RT 86 .H85 1988
Stress in the nursing
Humphrey, James Harry

121574

STRESS IN
THE NURSING PROFESSION

ABOUT THE AUTHOR

James H. Humphrey, Professor Emeritus at the University of Maryland, has taught courses for nurses at the University of Maryland School of Nursing and Walter Reed Hospital in Washington, D.C. He is the author of over 40 books and 200 articles and research reports. Nine of his most recent books have been in the area of stress.

STRESS IN
THE NURSING PROFESSION

By

JAMES H. HUMPHREY, ED.D.

Professor Emeritus
University of Maryland

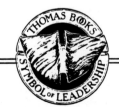

CHARLES C THOMAS • PUBLISHER
Springfield • Illinois • U.S.A.

Published and Distributed Throughout the World by

CHARLES C THOMAS • PUBLISHER

2600 South First Street

Springfield, Illinois 62794-9265

© *1988 by* CHARLES C THOMAS • PUBLISHER

ISBN 0-398-05441-X

Library of Congress Catalog Card Number: 87-33547

With THOMAS BOOKS *careful attention is given to all details of manufacturing and
design. It is the Publisher's desire to present books that are satisfactory as to their physical
qualities and artistic possibilities and appropriate for their particular use.* THOMAS
BOOKS *will be true to those laws of quality that assure a good name and good will.*

Printed in the United States of America

Q-R-3

Library of Congress Cataloging in Publication Data

Humphrey, James Harry, 1911-
    Stress in the nursing profession / by James H.
Humphrey.
        p. cm.
    Bibliography: p.
    Includes index.
    ISBN 0-398-05441-X
    1. Nurses—Job stress. 2. Stress (Psychology)
—Prevention. I. Title
    [DNLM: 1. Nursing—psychology. 2. Stress,
Psychological—prevention & control—nurses' in-
struction. WY 87 H926s]
RT86.H85   1988
610.73'01'9—dc19
DNLM/DLC   87-33547
for Library of Congress   CIP

PREFACE

THIS BOOK IS about the problems faced by nurses and the stress brought about by these problems. Although the book is for and about nurses and prospective nurses, it should be of interest to anyone in the medical profession who has any concern with nursing. It could also serve as a basic or supplementary text in college courses for nurses.

The introductory chapter presents a brief overview of the history and current status and trends in nursing. Chapter Two is concerned with nurses' concepts of stress and the following chapter provides information that nurses should have about stress.

In the fourth chapter emotional aspects of stress are discussed along with the extent to which nurses are involved in certain emotional patterns on the job. Chapter Five delineates causes of stress provided by nurses themselves, as well as how they try to deal with such stress.

Chapter Six deals with behavior modification as a stress-reducing technique for nurses. The discussion in Chapter Seven goes into detail regarding a stress management personal health regimen for nurses. The final chapter is concerned with how nurses can induce the relaxation response through such techniques as progressive relaxation, meditation, and biofeedback.

A book is seldom the product of an author alone. Admittedly, the author does most of the things concerned with actually putting a book together. However, it is almost always true that many individuals participate, at least indirectly, in some way before a book is finally "put to bed." This volume is no exception.

To acknowledge everyone personally would be practically impossible. For example, there was a large number of nurses who participated in my extensive survey in the acquisition of data which was pertinent to the book. I would like to express a debt of gratitude to them collectively for taking the time to provide this important information.

It is possible and practical, however, to cite certain individuals personally.

To the late Dr. Hans Selye (generally known as the "father of stress"), with whom I collaborated on certain aspects of stress research, I am most grateful for his inspiration in all of my writing on stress.

Also I wish to extend my thanks to two individuals who were kind enough to assist me with the distribution of the inquiry forms for my survey of nurses: Frances P. Cave, Primary Care Coordinator at the University of Maryland Health Center, and Flora B. Haus, Nursing Supervisor, The Alexandria Hospital, Alexandria, Virginia.

JAMES H. HUMPHREY

CONTENTS

STRESS IN
THE NURSING PROFESSION

CHAPTER ONE

INTRODUCTION

"ARE THE nation's nurses fed up?" This was the question posed by Oprah Winfrey when introducing her widely watched television program on August 6, 1987. The nurses on the program commented on what they referred to as "horror stories" that they and other nurses encounter almost daily on the job.

Among the distinguished panel of nurses was Echo Heron, author of the recently published *Intensive Care: The Story of a Nurse.*[4] In her book the author cites a provocative "job description" of the nurse:

> A nurse is a warrior against death and suffering, a technician of the highest degree, a mother, a sister, a best friend, a psychiatrist, a teacher, a magician, a sounding board, a secretary, a fortune teller, a politician, but most of all a loving human being who has chosen to give that love in one of the best ways you can.

Indeed, when nurses were first labeled "angels of mercy," they were suitably portrayed. In my own personal experience in teaching courses to undergraduate, graduate, and nurses in service, I found that the one characteristic that most of them had in common was that of *dedication and caring*. This despite the fact that, for the most part, they are overworked, underpaid, and in too many instances downright "put upon" in one way or another.

No question about it, the profession of nursing has travelled a strange and sometimes hazardous road in reaching its current status. The following brief summary highlights some of the aspects of the profession since its inception.

In the middle ages, nurses were nuns or women in secular orders of the church. The Augustinian sisters at the Hôtel Dieu in Paris, cooked, served meals, washed, and sewed for the sick. They cut hair, pared nails, gave enemas, and administered medicines prescribed by doctors.

3

In the eighteenth century, nursing in public hospitals was thought to be degrading, and doctors considered nurses to be little more than incompetent maids. (As we shall see in a later chapter, in modern times some nurses feel that physicians are stress-inducing factors for them.) In the yellow fever epidemic in Philadelphia in 1793, women convicts and other women of poor reputation served as hospital nurses.

Some reforms were begun in Kaiserwerth, Germany around the mid-nineteenth century when Theodor Fliedner, a Lutheran minister, and his wife set up a three-year training course for nurses. The girls learned housekeeping, cooking, and bookkeeping, served in hospital wards, and were taught the fundamentals of anatomy, physiology, and pharmacy.[5]

It was there that Florence Nightingale received the training that helped her to establish at St. Thomas's Hospital in London, the first school designed primarily to train nurses rather than to provide nursing services for the hospital. Similar schools were established in 1873 in New York City, New Haven, and Boston. Since then nursing has become one of the most important professions open to women (and to a lesser extent to men). Nursing candidates must prepare themselves through a rigorous course of study. Many nurses prepare themselves for specialized work, such as the care of newborn infants, maternity patients, the mentally ill, or for duties in the operating room.

Training for a career as a Registered Nurse can be met by various possibilities in terms of programs of study: a two-year course at a junior college, a three-year hospital course, or a four-year degree program at a college or university. More emphasis is being placed on a college education for nurses because greater knowledge is required to apply the latest methods of diagnosis and therapy. Training by any of the above methods includes both classroom study and actual hospital practice, and the graduate must still be examined and licensed by the state. This applies also to women in religious orders who train and work as nursing sisters. In addition to the duties in the hospital or in the home there are many fields open to the professional nurse, such as the Red Cross, military service, public health agencies, industry, teaching, and missionary work in remote areas of the world.[6]

In modern times there is a phenomenal shortage of nurses and this is due largely to the two factors of low salary and stress on the job. The vacancy rate for Registered Nurses in hospitals nationwide more than doubled in 1986 to 13.6 percent, according to a December 1986 survey by the American Hospital Association. Between 1979 and 1983, the rate was an all-time high of 14 percent but had dropped to 6.3 percent in September 1985.[2]

Severest shortages were in the Northeast United States, but shortages were reported in all of the 48 mainland states. It was estimated that, in 1981, of 1.4 million licensed Registered Nurses only half, or about 719,000 were full time nurses. In 1986, out of 1.5 million licensed Registered Nurses, one-third worked outside the hospital setting.[3]

The problem of stress in nursing has been well known for some time. In 1977, the National Institute of Occupational Safety and Health ranked 130 occupations by rate of admission to community mental health centers in Tennessee. The purpose was to determine the relative risk of psychological or stress-related disorders by occupation. Registered Nurses ranked 27th on the list. Licensed Practical Nurses ranked third, and Nurses' Aides were tenth.[1]

A portion of the content for this book was derived from my extensive survey of nurses. In this survey a random sample was selected from 40,000 nurses in the District of Columbia, Northern Virginia, and Maryland. The Humphrey Stress Inquiry Form (modified for nurses) and an accompanying letter of instructions were sent to each of the nurses in the sample. The responses were anonymous and of a self-reporting nature. Interest in the study was demonstrated by the high rate of return of 73 percent.

The range of ages of the nurses in the survey was 22 to 67 years with the average age being 39 years. Years of experience ranged from one year to 46 years for an average of 14 years of experience. The wide range of nursing specialities is reflected in the following partial list. (There may be some duplication because of different uses in terminology.)

1. Ambulatory Care
2. Bed Control
3. Chemical Dependency
4. Clinical
5. College Health
6. Community Health
7. Critical Care
8. Dialysis
9. Geriatrics
10. Inservice Education
11. Intensive Care

12. Labor and Delivery Room
13. Medical/Surgical
14. Nursing Administration
15. Obstetrics/Gynecology
16. Office Nursing
17. Operating Room
18. Progressive Care
19. Psychiatric
20. Recovery Room
21. Rehabilitation Nursing
22. School Health
23. Staff Nurse
24. Urgent Care
25. Women's Health

Although various estimates place the number of male nurses as high as two percent, none turned up in my sample.

In addition to answering items on the inquiry form, many of the nurse respondents made various interesting comments. Some representative examples of these follow:

> I wish you success in your study! If someone could show me how to at least decrease the stress in hospital nursing, I'd go back in a heartbeat and I think a lot of nurses feel that way — it sure would help the shortage. But it seems that today everyone is angry — hospital administrators, physicians, patients, their families — and the nursing staff always takes the blame and abuse. No one can work with all that anger!

> My nursing profession is a means to an end. It provides me the financial support for my continuing education and that of my children. My satisfaction is achieved apart from my career, primarily through my family and educational achievements.

> The bottom line is not enough nurses due to burnout, demands from families making the hours unrealistic, working weekends, etc. Other jobs with higher pay and less stress seem more appealing. The higher pay available in some cases for nurses now is not as attractive due to the unrealistic work assignments which are physically and emotionally exhausting and unsafe for the patients.

And finally on the need for a book such as this:

> I read a lot of articles on 'How to Relieve Stress' but not many pertain to nursing specifically.

REFERENCES

1. Colligan, M.J., M.J. Smith, and J.J. Hurrell. Occupational Incidence of Mental Health Disorders, *Journal of Human Stress,* 3, 1977.
2. Curran, C.R., A. Minnick, and J. Moss. Who Needs Nurses? *American Journal of Nursing,* 87, 1987.
3. Fewer Nurses, Growing Demand Seen, *American Medical News,* August 14, 1987.
4. Heron, Echo. *Intensive Care: The Story of a Nurse,* New York, Atheneum, 1987.
5. *The Modern Medical Encyclopedia,* Benjamin F. Miller (ed.), New York, Golden Press, 1965.
6. *The New Columbia Encyclopedia,* New York, Columbia University Press, 1975.

CHAPTER TWO

HOW STRESS IS PERCEIVED BY NURSES

SINCE THE term *stress* appears to mean so many different things to different people, I considered it appropriate to try to get some idea of nurses' concepts of it. This was accomplished by having my nurse respondents complete the following sentence: Stress is _____.

It is to be expected that there would be a rather wide variety of responses among nurses as far as their concepts of stress were concerned. In fact, "experts" themselves are not always in complete agreement as to its precise meaning (I will give a description of stress in the following chapter). My consideration of how nurses perceive stress focused on the number of times *key* words emerged in the responses. By identifying such key words it was felt that a more or less valid assessment of how nurses conceived of what stress means to them could be obtained. (See Table 1 — Note: In all instances where respondents could make more than one choice, the total percentages could go over 100 percent. This applies to other items in the inquiry form as well.)

Table 1
Percent of Time Certain Key Words Occurred
in Nurses' Concepts of Stress

Key Word	Percent of Time Occurring
Anxiety	32%
Emotion	19%
Tension	17%
Pressure	16%
Strain	12%
Frustration	10%
No Key Words	8%

In examining Table 1, attention of the reader is called to the fact that in all of the other populations I have studied the key word *pressure* appeared the most times, and at a rate of twice as many times as the second key word. These populations included teachers, psychiatrists, obstetricians, U.S. Congressmen and athletic coaches. In the population of nurses the key word *anxiety* occurred twice as many times as the key word *pressure*.

Anxiety. As noted, this was by far the most popular key word used by nurses in defining their concept of stress. This term is often used to mean the same thing as stress. In fact, some of the literature uses the expression "anxiety *or* stress," implying that they are one and the same thing. This can lead to the "chicken and egg" controversy; that is, is stress the cause of anxiety or is anxiety the cause of stress? Or, is it a reciprocal situation?

A basic literal meaning of the term anxiety is *uneasiness of the mind*. However, this simple generalization may be more complex than one might think. Even clinical psychologists who deal with this area sometimes have difficulty defining the term. Some consider it to be the reaction to a situation where we believe our well-being is endangered or threatened in some way. More specifically, others think of it as being closely associated with fear, and it is maintained that the fear can lead to anger, with the anger becoming guilt and finally if the guilt is not relieved, ending in a state of serious depression.

Some schools of thought contend that anxiety occurs when people are faced with more stress than they can handle. Although a certain amount of anxiety is normal and probably unavoidable, it can become a problem when it is inappropriate or out of proportion to a situation or when it interferes with normal activities. Ordinarily, it is suggested that excessive anxiety may be occurring when the following symptoms are noticed.

Irritability and tension
Insomnia
Demanding attitude
Loss of appetite
Restlessness
Headaches
Unwarranted concern about a physical ailment

Of course, these are also symptomatic of a variety of other types of disorders.

The following are some representative examples of how nurses used the word anxiety in their concept of stress.

Stress is:

The result of anxiety.

Anxiety caused by worry.

Those factors which create for the individual or that the individual creates which provide internal anxiety.

The feeling of anxiety I have over what events may happen to me in the future.

A state of anxiety created by having to cope with situations beyond my immediate control.

Anxiety produced by lack of skill, energy or time to do a job rewarding and beneficial to my patients.

Those occurrences and situations that cause me anxiety and a feeling of loss of control to some degree.

That feeling of anxiety due to increased responsibility.

Anxiety caused by racing thoughts of all that needs to be accomplished in too little time.

Any good or bad occurrence that increases anxiety.

Anxiety and responsibility you feel at work that affects you physically.

A feeling of anxiety and being overwhelmed.

Anxiety with a feeling of loss of control.

Mental and physical anxiety.

A cause of anxiety.

Anxiety which can cause a nurse not to be successful.

Emotion. The key word appearing second most frequently at 19 percent of the time was emotion. Since the terms *stress* and *emotion* are used interchangeably in the literature, consideration should be given to the meaning of the latter term. A description of emotion that I tend to like is one that views it as the response an individual makes when confronted with a situation for which he or she is unprepared or which he or she interprets as a possible source of gain or loss. For example, if an individual is confronted with a situation for which he or she may not have a satisfactory response, the emotional pattern of fear could result. Or, if one's desires are frustrated, the emotional pattern of anger may occur. Emotion, then, is not the state of stress itself but rather it is a stressor that can stimulate stress. (The subject of emotion will be discussed in greater detail in Chapter Four.)

In regard to their stress concept some nurses used the term emotion as follows.

Stress is:

A bad emotional experience.

Is concerned with emotional upset.

A situation which causes emotional outburst.

Emotion that influences one negatively.

Emotional reaction to negative influences in my environment.

A physical and emotional reaction to a real or anticipated occurrence.

A condition produced by lack of skill, energy, or time to do a job both rewarding emotionally and beneficial to my patients.

The way one reacts physically or emotionally to change.

Emotion induced by life experience.

Emotional response to danger.

A situation that influences you emotionally.

An uncomfortable level of demands on either my emotions, my mental abilities, my physical or social self.

Events that subject a person to an altered emotional state.

Tension. The key word appearing third most frequently at 17 percent of the time was tension. This term is often used in relation to stress. It is interesting to examine the entries used for the terms stress and tension in the *Education Index.* This bibliographical index of periodical educational literature records entries on these two terms as follows:

Stress (physiology)
Stress (psychology) see *Tension* (psychology)
Tension (physiology) see *Stress* (physiology)
Tension (psychology)

This indicates that there are physiological and psychological aspects of both stress and tension. However, articles in the periodical literature listed as "stress" articles seem to imply that stress is more physiologically-oriented and that tension is more psychologically-oriented. Thus, psychological stress and psychological tension could be interpreted to mean the same thing. The breakdown in this position is seen where there is another entry for tension concerned with *muscular* tension. The latter, of course, must be considered to have a physiological orientation. In the final analysis, the validity of these entries will depend upon the point of view of each individual. As we shall see later, the validity of this particular cataloging of these terms may possibly be at odds with a more specific meaning of the term.

The late Arthur Steinhaus,[2] a notable physiologist considered tensions as unnecessary or exaggerated muscle contractions, which could be accomplished by abnormally great or reduced activities of the internal organs. He viewed tensions in two frames of reference; first, as *physiologic* or *unlearned tensions*, and second, as *psychologic* or *learned tensions*. An example of the first, physiologic or unlearned tensions, would be "tensing" at bright lights or intense sounds. He considered psychologic or learned tensions as responses to stimuli that ordinarily do not involve muscular contractions, but that at sometime earlier in a person's experience were associated with a situation in which tension was a part of the normal response. In view of the fact that the brain connects any events that stimulate it simultaneously, it would appear to follow that, depending upon the unlimited kinds of personal experiences one might have, he or she may show tension to any and all kinds of stimuli. An example of psychologic or learned tension would be an inability to relax when riding in a car after experiencing or imagining too many automobile accidents.

In a sense, it may be inferred that physiologic or unlearned tensions are current and spontaneous, while psychologic or learned tensions may be latent as a result of a previous experience and may emerge at a later time. Although there may be a hairline distinction in the minds of some people, perhaps an essential difference between stress and tension is that the former is a physical and/or mental state concerned with wear and tear on the organism, while the latter is either a spontaneous or latent condition which can bring about this wear and tear.

Most often those nurses who used the word tension in expressing their concept of stress, did so in the following manner.

Stress is:

Tension that is sometimes useful and sometimes detrimental to the individual.
Tension from overwork.
Those conditions which create for one a feeling of tension.
Tension caused by a situation over which I have little or no control.
Mental or physical tension.
The feeling of increased tension due to demands.
Tension induced by work.
When I am overcome by tension.

A lot of tension at one time.
A combination of several unfavorable conditions that cause tension.
Tension that can cause stomach upset.

Pressure. Closing following tension was the word pressure at 16 percent of the time. The word pressure rarely appears in the literature on stress except when it is used in connection with blood pressure. It is interesting to note that the lead definition of the term in most standard dictionaries considers it in relation to the human organism by referring to pressure as "burden of physical and mental distress."

Some representative examples of how nurses used the word pressure in describing their concept of stress follow.

Stress is:

The result of pressure.
Pressure from job put on us by management, patients, visitors and
    staff.
Feeling of being overwhelmed, pressured and burned out, and a feel-
    ing that control over one's envrionment is being lost.
Pressure controlling the physical body and mental attitude.
Pressure to keep up physically during patient overload.
Pressure and responsibility felt at work.
Feeling overwhelmed and pressured with confused thinking.
Concerned with relieving the pressure you feel.
Constant pressure on mind and body.
The pressure of daily problems.
Pressure that is harmful to you.

Strain. This key word appeared 12 percent of the time. As we shall see later the word strain derives from the same Latin word as stress. This being the case, it would be easy to rationalize that stress and strain might be considered the same thing. In this regard, it is interesting to note that Paul J. Rosch,[1] President of the American Institute of Stress, has asserted that the late Hans Selye once complained to him that had his knowledge of English been more precise, he might have labeled his hypothesis the *strain concept*. In fact, Selye did encounter all sorts of problems when his research had to be translated into foreign languages. In the late 1940s, when Selye was invited to give a series of lectures at the College de France, the academicians there had a great deal of difficulty finding a suitable word or phrase to describe this new entity. Consequently, a new word had to be created. And so *le stress* was born, quickly followed by *el stress, der stress, lo stress,* with similar neologisms in Russian, Chinese, Japanese, and so forth.

The term strain tends to be used in connection with unusual tension in a muscle caused by overuse or because of a sudden unaccustomed movement. (A *strain* is a milder injury than a *sprain* in which ligaments around a joint are pulled or torn, and swelling occurs.)

Examples of how nurses used the word strain in describing stress are listed below.

Stress is:

Mental or physical strain.
A mental or physical strain on a person's coping mechanisms, on the
    body's ability to adapt to change.
The strain resulting from situations encountered in everyday living.
A strain on your health.
Strain brought about because of worry.
Strain from overwork.
Strain caused by unknown sources.

Frustration. This key word appeared ten percent of the time when nurses indicated their concept of stress. When stress is induced as a result of the individual's not being able to meet his or her needs (basic demands) and satisfy desires (wants or wishes), frustration or conflict results. Frustration occurs when a need is not met, and conflict results when choices must be made between nearly equally attractive alternatives or when basic emotional forces oppose one another. In the emotionally healthy person, the degree of frustration is ordinarily in proportion to the intensity of the need or desire. That is, he or she will objectively observe and evaluate a situation to ascertain whether a solution is possible, and if so, what solution would best enable him or her to achieve the fulfillment of needs or desires.

Some examples of how nurses used the term frustration follow.

Stress is:

A feeling of frustration caused by having too much to do in too short
    a time.
That feeling of increased frustration due to increased responsibility.
Frustration because of not being able to be of more help to patients.
Feeling of frustration if you do a poor job.
The feeling of frustration you get when things are not going well.
Frustration caused by a mental state.

Frustration that uses up your energy.

In eight percent of the cases none of the above key words were used by nurses in describing stress. Some of these statements follow.

Stress is:

An internal force created by real, or imagined unmet needs.

Being stretched like a rubber band.

The feeling of impending danger to complete life threatening demands.

A feeling of being out of control with no positive direction to turn to.

A heavy caseload of patients who are very sick, very demanding and who require you to work with little resources and time.

When you have reached your maximum stimulation threshold.

Where level of coverage and competency is overtaxed to becoming dangerous for patient and nurse.

Being overworked, underpaid and not respected for your abilities.

In summarizing the responses of nurses, two rather interesting bits of information emerged. First, there were relatively few who saw any aspect of stress as positive. That is, the responses were predominantly of a nature that conceived stress as always being undesirable with little or no positive effects. (Incidentally, in the following chapter, I will discuss eustress and distress, considered to be good and bad forms of stress.) Second, in a large percentage of the cases nurses' concepts of stress tended to focus on the *stressor* rather than on the condition of stress itself. This would appear to be natural since it has been only in relatively recent years that literature on the subject of stress has become more plentiful in terms of describing what it is and how it affects the human organism. At any rate, the responses of nurses about their concepts of stress provided certain important guidelines in preparing content for the book. Because of this, the collection of such data was a worthwhile undertaking; and, in fact, some nurses said that filling out this item as well as others on the inquiry form caused them to think more about it.

REFERENCES

1. Rosch, Paul J. In Human Stress: Current Selected Research, Volume 1. James H. Humphrey (ed.), New York, AMS Press, Inc.
2. Steinhaus, Arthur. *Toward an Understanding of Health and Physical Education*, Dubuque, Iowa, Wm. C. Brown Publisher, 1963.

CHAPTER THREE

INFORMATION ABOUT STRESS
FOR NURSES

A S MENTIONED previously, my extensive survey of nurses tended to show that nurses' concepts of stress, for the most part, focused on stressors rather than on the condition of stress itself. In fact, although the respondents felt that their work environment was a stressful one, at the same time many of them professed that their knowledge about the stress concept is somewhat limited. For this reason it seems appropriate to provide some information about stress for nurses, and the present chapter is devoted to that subject. An attempt will be made to present a relatively simplified discussion about a rather complex and complicated phenomenon.

THE MEANING OF STRESS

There is no solid agreement regarding the derivation of the term *stress*. For example, some sources suggest that the term is derived from the Latin word *stringere*, meaning "to bind tightly." Other sources contend that the term derives from the French word *destresse* (anglicized to *distress*), and suggest that the prefix "dis" was eventually eliminated due to slurring, as in the case of the word *because* sometimes becoming 'cause.

A common generalized literal description of the term stress is a "constraining force of influence." When applied to the human organism, this could be interpreted to mean the extent to which the body can withstand a given force or influence. In this regard one of the most often quoted description of stress is that of Hans Selye who described it as the "nonspecific response of the body to any demand made upon it."[14] This

17

means that stress involves a mobilization of the bodily resources in response to some sort of stimulus. These responses can include various physical and chemical changes in the organism. This description of stress could be extended by saying that it involves demands that tax and/ or exceed the resources of the human organism. This means that stress not only involves these bodily responses, but that it also involves wear and tear on the organism brought about by these responses. In essence, stress can be considered as any factor acting internally or externally that makes it difficult to adapt and that induces increased effort on the part of a person to maintain a state of equilibrium within himself and with his external environment.

THEORIES OF STRESS

It should be mentioned that it is not the intent to get into a highly technical discourse on the complex and complicated aspects of stress. However, there are certain basic understandings that need to be taken into account, and this requires the use of certain technical terms. For this reason, it appears appropriate to provide an "on-the-spot" glossary of terms used in the discussion to follow.

ACTH—(AdrenoCorticoTropic Hormone) secreted by the pituitary gland. It influences the function of the adrenals and other glands in the body.

ADRENALIN—A hormone secreted by the medulla of the adrenal glands.

ADRENALS—Two glands in the upper posterior part of the abdomen that produce and secrete hormones. They have two parts, the outer layer, called the *cortex* and the inner core called the *medulla*.

CORTICOIDS—Hormones produced by the adrenal cortex, an example of which is *cortisone*.

ENDOCRINE—Glands that secrete their hormones into the blood stream.

HORMONE—A chemical produced by a gland, secreted into the blood stream, and influencing the function of cells or organs.

HYPOTHALAMUS—The primary activator of the autonomic nervous system, it plays a central role in translating neurological stimuli into endocrine processes during stress reactions.

PITUITARY—An endocrine gland located at the base of the brain about the size of a pea. It secretes important hormones, one of which is the *ACTH* hormone.

THYMUS—A ductless gland that is considered a part of the endo-crine gland system, located behind the upper part of the breast bone.

Although there are various theories of stress, one of the better known ones and one to which most others are anchored, is that of Hans Selye. I have already given Selye's description of stress as the "nonspecific re-sponse of the body to any demand made upon it." The physiological pro-cesses and the reaction involved in Selye's stress model is known as the *General Adaptation Syndrome* and consists of three stages of *alarm reaction, re-sistance stage,* and the *exhaustive stage.*

In the first stage (alarm reaction), the body reacts to the stressor and causes the hypothalamus to produce a biochemical "messenger" which in turn causes the pituitary gland to secrete ACTH into the blood. This hormone then causes the adrenal gland to discharge adrenalin and other corticoids. This causes shrinkage of the thymus with an influence on heart rate, blood pressure, and the like. It is during the alarm stage that the resistance of the body is reduced.

In the second stage, *resistance* develops if the stressor is not too pro-nounced. Body adaptation develops to fight back the stress or possibly avoid it, and the body begins to repair damage, if any.

The third stage of *exhaustion* occurs if there is a long-continued expo-sure to the same stressor. The ability of adaptation is eventually ex-hausted and the signs of the first state (alarm reaction) reappear. Selye contended that our adaptation resources are limited, and, when they be-come irreversible, the result is death.

As mentioned previously, Selye's stress model, which places emphasis upon "nonspecific" responses, has been widely recognized. However, the nonspecific nature of stress has been questioned by some. In this con-nection, reference is made to the brilliant research of John W. Mason,[10] a former president of the American Psychosomatic Society. His findings tend to support the idea that there are other hormones involved in stress in addition to those of the pituitary-adrenal system. Mason's data sug-gest that psychological stressors activate other endocrine systems beside those activated by physiological stressors such as cold, electric shock, and the like.

As in the case of all research, the search for truth will continue and more and more precise and sophisticated procedures will emerge in the scientific study of stress. Current theories will be more critically appraised and evaluated, and other theories will continue to be advanced. In the meantime, there is abundant evidence to support the notion that stress in modern society is a most serious threat to the well-being of man if not controlled, and of course the most important factor in such control is man himself.

REACTIONS TO STRESS

There are various ways in which reactions to stress can be classified, and, in any kind of classification, there will be some degree of unavoidable overlapping. In the classification here I arbitrarily suggest two broad classifications as *physiological* and *behavioral*.

Physiological Reactions

Although all individuals do not always react in the same way *physiologically* as far as stress is concerned, the following generalized list suggests some of the more or less standard body reactions.

1. Rapid beating of the heart, which has sometimes been described as "pounding of the heart." We have all experienced this reaction at one time or another as a result of great excitement, or as a result of being afraid.
2. Perspiration, which is mostly of the palms of the hands, although there may be profuse sweating in some individuals at various other parts of the body.
3. The blood pressure rises, which may be referred to as a hidden reaction because the individual is not likely to be aware of it.
4. The pupils of the eyes may dilate, and, again the individual will not necessarily be aware of it.
5. The stomach seems to "knot up" and we tend to refer to this as "feeling a lump in the pit of the stomach." This, of course, can have a negative influence on digestion.
6. Sometimes individuals experience difficulty in swallowing, which is often characterized as a "lump in the throat."
7. There may be a "tight" feeling in the chest and when the stressful condition is relieved one may refer to it as "getting a load off my chest."

What these various bodily reactions mean is that the organism is gearing up for a response to a stressor. This phenomenon is called the *fight or flight* response and was first described as an *emergency* reaction by Walter B. Cannon,[3] the famous Harvard University Professor of Physiology a good many years ago. The fight or flight response prepares us for action in the same way that it did for prehistoric man when he was confronted with an enemy. His responses were decided on the basis of the particular situation, such as fighting an opponent for food or fleeing from an animal that provided him with an overmatched situation. In modern times, with all of the potentially stressful conditions that provoke a fight or flight response, modern man uses these same physiological responses to face up to these kinds of situations. However, today, we generally do not need to fight physically (although we might feel like it sometimes), or run from wild animals, but our bodies still react with the same fight or flight response. Physiologists point out that we still need this means of self-preservation occasionally, but not in response to the emotional traumas and anxieties of modern living.

Behavioral Reactions

In discussing behavioral reactions, it should be mentioned again that various degrees of unavoidable overlapping may occur between these reactions and physiological reactions. Although behavioral reactions are, for the most part, physically-oriented, they are likely to involve more overt manifestations than are provoked by the physiological reactions. For purposes of this discussion I will consider *behavior* to mean anything that one does as a result of some sort of stimulation.

A person under stress will function with a behavior that is different from ordinary behavior. I will arbitrarily subclassify these as: (1) *counter* behavior (sometimes referred to as defensive behavior), (2) *dysfunctional* behavior, and (3) *overt* behavior (sometimes referred to as expressive behavior).

In **Counter Behavior**, a person will sometimes take action that is intended to counteract the stressful situation. An example is an individual taking a defensive position; that is, a person practicing an "on-the-spot" relaxation technique, but at the same time, being unaware of it. He may take a deep breath and silently "count to ten" before taking action, if any.

Dysfunctional Behavior means that a person will react in a manner that demonstrates impaired or abnormal functioning, which results in a lower level of skill performance than he is ordinarily capable of accomplishing. There may be changes in the normal speech patterns, and there may be a temporary loss of memory. Many of us have experienced this at one time or another due to a stress-inducing situation, with a "mental block" causing some degree of frustration while we attempt to get back on the original train of thought.

Overt Behavior involves such reactions as distorted facial expressions (e.g., tics and twitches and biting the lip). There appears to be a need for a person to move about, and thus, pacing around is characteristic of this condition. Incidentally, there is a point of view that suggests that overt behavior in the form of activity is preferable for most individuals in most stressful situations, and can be highly effective in reducing threat and distress.

In fact, various authentic pronouncements have been made that support the idea that instant activity can be beneficial. For example, Reuven Gal and Richard Lazarus[6] report that being engaged in activity — rather than remaining passive — is preferable and can be highly effective in reducing threat and distress. Lazarus[9] has also maintained that a person may alter his or her psychological and physiological stress reactions in a given situation simply by taking action, and this in turn, affects his or her appraisal of the situation, thereby ultimately altering the stress reaction.

CLASSIFICATIONS OF STRESS

The difficulty encountered in attempting to devise a foolproof classification system for the various kinds of stress should be obvious. The reason for this, of course, lies in the fact that it is practically impossible to fit a given type of stress into one exclusive category because of the possibilities of overlapping. However, an attempt will be made to do so, and, as mentioned before, any such classification on my part is purely arbitrary. Others may wish to make different classifications than those used here and, in the absence of anything resembling standardization, it is their prerogative to do so. With this idea in mind, some general classifications of stress that will be dealt with in the following discussions are (1) desirable and undesirable stress, (2) physical stress, (3) psychological stress, and (4) social stress. It should be understood that this does not exhaust the possibilities of various kinds of stress classifications. That is, this particular listing is not necessarily theoretically complete, but for my purposes should suffice.

Desirable and Undesirable Stress

The classic comment by Selye that "stress is the spice of life" sums up the idea that stress can be desirable as well as devastating. He went on to say that the only way one could avoid stress would be to never do anything and that certain kinds of activities have a beneficial influence in keeping the stress mechanism in good shape. Certainly, the human organism needs to be taxed in order to function well, and it is a well-known physiological fact that muscles will soon atrophy if not subjected to sufficient use.

At one time or another most of us have experienced "butterflies in the stomach" when faced with a particularly challenging situation. Thus, it is important that we understand that stress is a perfectly normal human state and that the organism is under various degrees of stress in those conditions which are related to happiness as well as those concerned with sadness.

In the literature, undesirable stress may be referred to as *distress*. It is interesting to note that Selye referred to the pleasant or healthy kind of stress as "eustress," and to the unpleasant or unhealthy kind as "distress."

I have mentioned some of the desirable features of stress, but like any factor involving the human organism, most anything in excess is not good for it. Of course, this holds true for abnormal amounts of stress. When stress becomes prolonged and unrelenting, and thus chronic, it can result in very serious trouble.

It has been suggested that what we ordinarily refer to as *aging* may be nothing more than the sum total of all the scars left by the stress of life. This could be the reason why some comparatively young persons who are constantly under stress may "look old for their years." In the final analysis, the recommendation is not necessarily to avoid stress, but to keep it from becoming a chronic condition.

Although both "good" stress and "bad" stress reactions place specific demands for resources on the body, does this mean that good stress is "safe" and bad stress "dangerous?" Two prominent psychologists, Israel Posner and Lewis Leitner,[13] have some interesting suggestions in this regard. They feel that two psychological variables, *predictability* and *controllability* play an important role.

It can be reasoned that *predictable* pain and discomfort is less stressful because under this condition a person is said to be capable of learning when it is safe to "lower his guard" and relax. Since periods of impending pain are clearly signaled, the person can safely relax at times when the warning signal is absent. These periods of psychological safety seem to insulate individuals from harmful effects of stress. Obviously, persons receiving unsignaled pain have no way of knowing when it is safe to relax and thus are more likely to develop serious health problems as a result of the chronic psychological stress.

The second psychological variable, *controllability* of environmental stressors, which is closely related to coping behavior, also plays a major part in determining stress effects. The ability to control painful events may insulate individuals from experiencing damaging stress effects. However, such coping behavior is beneficial only if a person is given a feedback signal which informs him that the coping response was successful in avoiding an impending stressor. Without the feedback of success, active coping behavior, as such, may increase stress effects since it calls upon the energy reserves of the body and leaves it in a state of chronic stress.

The research on predictability and controllability of stressful events may help answer why it is that people who seek out stressful and challenging activities do not appear to develop stress illnesses from this form of stress. In contrast, when essentially similar body reactivity is produced by "bad" stress, then stress-related illnesses can be the result. Perhaps "good" stress does not produce illness because typically the events associated with it are planned in advance (they are predictable) or otherwise scheduled or integrated (they are controlled) into the individual's life. However, even activities which are generally considered to be pleasant and exciting (good stress) can produce illness if the individual is not forewarned or has little control over the events. And unpleasant events (bad stress) may result in stress-related illness because they generally come without warning and cannot be controlled.

In closing this section of the chapter, I should mention that some persons have taken the middle ground on this subject by saying that stress is not good nor bad, indicating that the effect of stress is not determined by the stress itself but how it is viewed and handled. That is, we either handle stress properly or we allow it to influence us negatively and thus become victims of undesirable stress.

Physical Stress

In discussing physical stress, it might be well to differentiate between the two terms *physical* and *physiological*. The former should be considered a broad term and can be described as "pertaining to or relating to the body." On the other hand, the term *physiological* is concerned with what the organs of the body do in relation to each other. Thus, physical stress could be conceived with unusual and excessive physical exertion, as well as certain physiological conditions brought about by some kind of stress.

Although there are many kinds of physical stress, they can be divided into two general types. One is referred to as *emergency* stress and the other as *continuing* stress. In emergency stress the previously described physiological reactions take place. That is, when an emergency arises such as bodily injury, hormones are discharged into the blood stream. This involves increase in heart rate, rise in blood pressure, and dilation of the blood vessels in the muscles to prepare themselves for immediate use of the energy that is generated.

In continuing stress the body reaction is more complicated. The physiological involvement is the same, but more and more hormones continue to be produced, the purpose of which is to increase body resistance. In cases where the stress is excessive, such as an extensive third degree burn, a third phase in the form of exhaustion of the adrenal glands can develop, sometimes culminating in fatality.

I have said that physical stress can be concerned with unusual and excessive exertion. This can be shown in a general way by performing an experiment involving some more or less mild physical exertion. First, try to find your resting pulse. This can be done by placing your right wrist, palm facing you, in your left hand. Now, bring the index and middle fingers of your left hand around the wrist and press lightly until you feel the beat of your pulse. Next, time this beat for ten seconds and then multiply this figure by six. This will give you your resting pulse rate per minute. For example, if you counted 12 beats in ten seconds, your resting pulse is 72 beats per minute. The next step is to engage in some physical activity. Stand and balance yourself on one foot. Hop up and down on this foot for a period of about 30 seconds, or less if it is too strenuous. Then, take your pulse again in the same manner suggested above. You will find that, as a result of this activity, your pulse rate will be elevated above your resting pulse. Even with this small amount of physical exertion, the body was adjusting to cope with it, as evidenced by the rise in pulse rate. This was noticable to you; however, other things such as a slight rise in blood pressure were likely involved and of which you were not aware.

Psychological Stress

The main difference between physical stress and psychological stress is that the former involves a real situation, while psychological stress is more concerned with foreseeing or imagining an emergency situation. As an example, a vicarious experience of danger may be of sufficient intensity to cause muscle tension and elevate the heart rate.

It has been clearly demonstrated that prolonged and unrelenting nervous tension developing from psychological stress can result in mental anguish, which in turn can cause various serious problems.

It should be mentioned that physiological and psychological conceptions of stress have evolved independently within their respective fields. Attempts are now being made to integrate these two conceptions. One writer on the subject, Anis Mikhail[11] has proposed the following holistic definition of stress for the purpose of emphasizing the continuity between psychological and physiological theorizing: "Stress is a state which arises from an actual or perceived demand-capability imbalance in the organism's vital adjustment actions, and which is partially manifested by a nonspecific response."

Social Stress

Human beings are social beings. They do things together. They play together. They work together for the benefit of society. They have fought together in time of national emergency in order to preserve the kind of society in which they believe. This means that life involves a constant series of social interactions. These interactions involve a two-way street, in that the individual has some sort of impact upon society, and in turn, society has an influence upon the individual. There are obviously many levels of social stress in life situations. For example, economic conditions and other social problems have been found to be very stressful situations for many people. Specifically, there are numerous possibiliies for social stress in the nursing situation. Nurses must interact with various persons such as patients, family members of patients, and physicians along with a host of others.

Negative attitudes about social interactions will almost always generate hard feelings and hostility among groups, making for more stressful conditions for all concerned. Also, a neutral or *laissez faire* attitude often degenerates into one of tolerance and, as such, can become almost as devastating as a negative attitude. In fact, the development of an "I don't care" attitude can often make life intolerable and bring about stress. In the final analysis, people themselves hold the key to the avoidance of undesirable social stress in any kind of environment, and good social relationships are most likely to be obtained if one assumes a positive attitude in such relationships.

CAUSES OF STRESS

A fair question to raise might be: What doesn't cause stress? I mention this because most human environments and society as a whole are now seen as stress-inducing to some degree. In recent years so many causes of cancer have been identified that many persons have almost come to the conclusion that "everything causes cancer." Perhaps the same could be said of stress. Because it seems to have reached "epidemic" proportions, it is easy to believe that "everything causes stress."

In the past decade or so a number of researchers have studied certain *life events* as causes of stress. They have attempted to find out what kinds of health problems are associated with various events, normal and abnormal, that occur to people either in the normal course of events or as a result of some sort of misfortune. One of the best known studies is that of Holmes and Rahe.[7] Following is a list of their ten most serious life events causing stress.

1. Death of a spouse
2. Divorce
3. Marital separation
4. Jail term
5. Death of a close family member
6. Personal injury or illness
7. Marriage
8. Fired at work
9. Marital reconciliation
10. Retirement

As important as life events scales are as a means of detecting causes of stress, they are not without their critics. Some specialists feel that rather than life events, a better measure is that which is concerned with day-to-day problems. Prominent in this regard is Richard Lazarus[8] the distinguished stress researcher at the University of California at Berkeley. He and his associates collected data on a number of populations on what he identifies as daily "hassles." Following is the list of hassles for one of these populations — 100 white, middle-class, middle-aged men and women.

1. Concern about weight

2. Health of a family member
3. Rising prices of common goods
4. Home maintenance
5. Too many things to do
6. Misplacing or losing things
7. Yard work or outside maintenance
8. Property, investment, or taxes
9. Crime
10. Physical appearance

Nurses, because of the very nature of their work, are susceptible to many stress inducing factors, and these factors will be dealt with in detail later.

EFFECTS OF STRESS

The same line of thought that prompted my comment: "everything causes stress," could be applied with the assertion that "stress causes everything." For example, Kenneth Pelletier[12] has reported that a tragic consequence is that stress-related psychological and physiological disorders have become the number one social and health problem in the last few years, and, further, that most standard medical textbooks attribute anywhere from 50 to 80 percent of all diseases to stress-related origins.

Recently I reviewed the literature by various medical authorities and found that among various other conditions, the following in some way could be stress-related: diabetes, cirrhosis of the liver, high blood pressure, peptic ulcer, migraine headaches, multiple sclerosis, herpes, lung disease, injury due to accidents, mental breakdown, cancer, and coronary heart disease.

One of the more recent findings has been that there is evidence linking stress and the body's ability to fight disease. Some studies suggest the possibility of immune-system malfunction under stress by comparing the infection-fighting capability of white blood cells taken from normal and severely stressed individuals.

PERSONALITY AND STRESS

Before discussing personality as it pertains to stress, let me comment on my own idea of personality. Ordinarily, personality is often dealt with only in terms of the psychological aspect. I like to think of it in terms of the *total* personality. I view this total personality as consisting of physical, social, emotional, and intellectual aspects. This conforms more or less with what is becoming one rather common description of personality — "existence as a person" — and this should be interpreted to mean the *whole* person.

Although there might be general agreement that personality can influence the way individuals handle stress, there is much less agreement regarding personality as a causal factor in disease. One specific example of this is the difference in opinion regarding the extent to which certain types of personality are associated with heart disease as a result of stress. A case in point is the position taken by Friedman and Rosenman.[5] They have designated a Type A behavior and a Type B behavior. A person with type A behavior tends to be aggressive, ambitious, competitive, and puts pressure on himself in getting things done. An individual with Type B behavior is more easygoing, relaxed, and tends not to put pressure on himself. With regard to these two types of behavior Friedman and Rosenman state: "In the absence of Type A Behavior Patterns, coronary heart disease almost never occurs before 70 years of age, regardless of the fatty food eaten, the cigarettes smoked, or the lack of exercise, but when this behavior pattern is present, coronary heart disease can easily erupt in one's thirties or forties."

This point of view has come under challenge by some, the main point of contention being that there is little in the way of solid objective scientific evidence to support the hypothesis. In fact, at one American Heart Association forum for science writers it was reported that scientific studies fail to show that stress causes heart attacks.[2] (Incidentally, it is interesting that many heart specialists have noted that death from heart disease is on a downward trend and may be expected to continue. They credit this, among other things, to diet, control of high blood pressure, and particularly to exercise.)

It is also interesting to note that at a recent special symposium on the interactions between the heart and brain at an American Psychiatric Association meeting,[1] Rosenman reported that a 22-year research project found that Type A's were twice as likely as B's to develop coronary heart disease. In addition, however, the highly competitive nature found in Type A people increases the likelihood that important warning signs of heart disease — such as chest pains — will be denied. It is maintained that Type A's also survive better than Type B's, and it is speculated that this may have something to do with Type A people's adeptness at denial.

This is to say that once a heart attack has occurred, Type A people tend to deny their symptoms, and therefore they may be better at suppressing the health anxieties that often accompany recovery from a heart attack. According to Rosenman, with less anxiety there is less adrenalin release and a greater feeling of control over one's life.

As far as nurses are concerned, research has shown that over 82 percent of one group of 65 nurses considered themselves to be Type A. Oftentimes they:

1. Engage in races against the clock and try to care for more and more patients on each shift.
2. Work double shifts with the intent of denying their limits.
3. Talk on the phone or to visitors and chart at the same time.
4. Measure their worth by the number of patients bathed, examined, interviewed, resuscitated, or, above all, "cured."
5. Resist innovation because it "slows things down."
6. View their peers as competitors, turning conferences into occasions for "one-upping" another or interpreting a simple offer to help as a slur on their competence.[4]

REFERENCES

1. Annual meeting of the American Psychiatric Association, Dallas, Texas, May 1985.
2. Auerbach, Stuart. Doctors Say Studies Fail to Prove That Stress Causes Heart Attacks, *Washington Post*, January 22, 1975.
3. Cannon, Walter B. *The Wisdom of the Body*, New York, W.W. Norton, 1932.
4. Cronin-Stubbs, D. and B. Velsor-Friedrich. Professional and Personal Stress, *Nurse Leadership*, April, 1981.
5. Friedman, Myer and Ray H. Rosenman. *Type A Behavior and Your Heart*, New York, Alfred A. Knopf, Inc., 1974.
6. Gal, Reuven and Richard S. Lazarus. The Role of Activity in Anticipating and Confronting Stressful Situations, *Journal of Human Stress*, December, 1975.
7. Holmes, T.H. and R.H. Rahe. The Social Adjustment Rating Scale, *Journal of Psychomatic Research*, 11: 1967.
8. Lazarus, Richard S. Little Hassles Can Be Hazardous to Your Health, *Psychology Today*, July, 1981.
9. Lazarus, Richard S. The Self-Regulation of Emotion, In *Parameters of Emotion*, L. Levy (ed.), New York, Raven Press, 1975.
10. Mason, John W., et al, Selectivity of Corticosteroids and Catecholamine Responses to Various Natural Stimuli, *Psychopathology of Human Adaptations*, New York, Plenum Publishing Co., 1976.

11. Mikhail, Anis. Stress: A Psychophysiological Conception, *Journal of Human Stress*, June, 1981.
12. Pelletier, Kenneth R. *Mind As Healer, Mind As Slayer*, Dell Publishing Company, Inc., 1977.
13. Posner, Israel and Lewis A. Leitner. Eustress vs. Distress: Determination by Predictability and Controllability of the Stressor, Stress, *The Official Journal of the International Institute of Stress and Its Affiliates*, Vol. 2, No. 2, Summer, 1981.
14. Selye, Hans. *Stress Without Distress*, New York, Signet New American Library, 1975.

CHAPTER FOUR

EMOTIONAL ASPECTS OF NURSING

IN INTRODUCING the subject of emotion, we are confronted with the fact that, for many years, it has been a difficult concept to define, and, in addition, there have been many changing ideas and theories as far as the study of emotions is concerned. Obviously, it is not the purpose of a book of this nature to attempt to go into any great depth on a subject that has been one of the most intricate undertakings of psychology for many years. However, a general overview of the subject appears to be in order to help the reader have a clearer understanding of the emotional aspect of nursing, particularly to its involvement in stress.

Emotional stress can be brought about by the stimulus of any of the emotional patterns. For example, the emotional pattern of anger can be stimulated by such factors as the thwarting of one's wishes, or a number of cumulative irritations. Response to such stimuli can be either *impulsive* or *inhibited*. An impulsive expression of anger is one that is directed against an object or a person. Inhibited expressions of anger are kept under control and may be manifested by such overt behaviors as skin flushing.

Generally speaking, emotional patterns can be placed in the two broad categories of *pleasant* and *unpleasant* emotions. Pleasant emotional patterns include such things as joy, affection, happiness, and love — in the broad sense, while included among the unpleasant emotional patterns are anger, sorrow, jealousy, fear and worry — an imaginary form of fear.

It is interesting to note that a good proportion of the literature is devoted to emotions that are unpleasant. It has been found that, in most basic psychology books, much more space is given to such emotional patterns as fear, hate, and guilt, than to such pleasant emotional patterns as love, sympathy, and contentment.

At one time or another most nurses have manifested emotional behavior as well as ordinary behavior. Differences in the structure of the organism and in the environment will largely govern the degree to which a nurse expresses emotional behavior. Moreover, it has been suggested that the pleasantness or unpleasantness of an emotion seems to be determined by its strength or intensity, by the nature of the situation arousing it, and by the way a nurse perceives or interprets the situation.

The ancient Greeks identified emotions with certain organs of the body. In general, sorrow was expressed from the heart (a broken heart); jealousy was associated with the liver; hate with the gall bladder; and anger with the spleen. I make this historical reference because in modern times we take into account certain conduits between the emotions and the body. These are by way of the *nervous* system and the *endocrine* system. That part of the nervous system principally concerned with the emotions is the *autonomic* nervous system, which controls functions such as the heart beat, blood pressure and digestion. When there is a stimulus of any of the emotional patterns, these two systems activate in the manner explained previously. By way of illustration, if the emotional pattern of fear is stimulated, the heartbeat accelerates, breathing is more rapid, and the blood pressure is likely to rise. Energy fuel is discharged into the blood from storage in the liver, which causes the blood sugar level to rise. These, along with other bodily functions serve to prepare one to cope with the condition caused by the fear. The person then reacts with the fight or flight response that was discussed previously.

When we attempt to evaluate the emotional aspect of personality, we encounter various degrees of difficulty, because of certain uncontrollable factors. Included among some of the methods used for attempting to measure emotional responses are the following.

1. Blood pressure: It rises when one is under some sort of emotional stress.
2. Blood sugar analysis: Under stressful conditions, more sugar enters the blood stream.
3. Galvanic skin response: Similar to the lie detector technique, and measurements are recorded in terms of perspiration on the palms of the hands.
4. Heart rate: Emotional stress causes it to elevate.

These measures, as well as others that have been used by investigators of human emotion, have various and perhaps limited degrees of validity. In attempting to assess emotional reactivity, we often encounter the problem of the extent to which we are dealing with a purely physiological response or a purely emotional response. For example, one's heart rate would be elevated by taking some sort of physical exercise. It could likewise be elevated when a nurse is in an emotional state during a critical situation. Thus, in this illustration, the elevation of heart rate could be caused for different reasons, the first being physiological and the second emotional. Then, too, the type of emotional pattern is not identified by the measuring device. A joy response and an anger response will likely show the same or nearly the same rise in heart rate. These are some of the reasons why it is most difficult to arrive at a high degree of objectivity in studying the emotional aspect of personality.

FACTORS CONCERNED WITH EMOTIONAL STABILITY

Nursing involves various kinds of experiences that are characterized by the necessity to adjust. It could be said that normal behavior is the result of successful adjustment, and abnormal behavior results from unsuccessful adjustment. The degree of adjustment that any nurse achieves depends upon how adequately she is able to satisfy basic needs and to fulfill desires within the framework of the environment and the pattern or ways dictated by the particular nursing situation.

As mentioned before, stress may be considered as any factor acting internally or externally that renders adaptation difficult, and which induces increased effort on the part of the person to maintain a state of equilibrium within himself or herself and with the environment. When stress is induced as a result of the individual's not being able to meet his or her needs (basic demands) and satisfy desires (wants and wishes), *frustration* and *conflict* result. As mentioned in Chapter Two, frustration occurs when a need is not met, and conflict results when choices must be made between nearly equally attractive alternatives or when basic emotional forces oppose one another. In the emotionally healthy person, the degree of frustration is ordinarily in proportion to the intensity of the need or desire. That is, one will objectively observe and evaluate the situation to ascertain whether a solution is possible, and if so, what solution would best enable one to achieve the fulfillment of needs or desires. However, every person has a *zone of tolerance* or limits for emotional stress within which he or she normally operates. If the stress becomes considerably greater than the tolerance level, or if the individual has not learned to cope with his or her problems and objectively and intelligently solve them, some degree of maladjustment possibly can result.

It could be said that the major difference between you, as a normal person, and a criminal confined to prison is that you have the ability to control your emotional impulses to a greater degree than such a person. Perhaps many of us at one time or another have experienced the same kinds of emotions that have led the abnormal individual to commit violence, but we have been able to hold our powerful and violent emotions in check. This may be an extreme example, but it should suggest something of the importance of emotional control in modern society.

An important aspect of controlling the emotions is becoming able to function effectively and intelligently in an emotionally charged situation. Success in most life situations—and particularly in the nursing profession—hinges upon this ability. Extremes of emotional upset must be avoided if a nurse is to be able to think and act effectively on the job.

It is sometimes helpful to visualize your emotions as being forces within you that are in a struggle for power with your mind as to which is to control you, your reason, or your emotions. Oftentimes, our basic emotions are blind and unconcerned with the welfare of other people, or sometimes, even with our own welfare. Emotional stability has to do with gaining increased mastery over our emotions—not, of course, eliminating them—so that we may behave as intelligent and civilized human beings.

In order to pursue a sensible course in our efforts to acquire desired emotional stability, there are certain factors that need to be taken into account. Some of these factors are the subject of the ensuing discussion.

Those factors concerned with emotional stability that need to be considered are: (1) characteristics of emotionality, (2) emotional arousals and reactions, and (3) factors that influence emotionality.

Characteristics of Emotionality

There are variations in how long emotions last. A child's emotions may last for a few minutes or less and then terminate rather abruptly. The child gets it "out of his system" so to speak by expressing it outwardly. In contrast, adult emotions may be long and drawn out. As children get older, expressing the emotions by overt action is encumbered by certain social restraints. This is to say that what might be socially acceptable at one age level is not necessarily so at another. This may be a reason for some children developing *moods*, which in a sense are states of emotion drawn out over a period of time and expressed slowly. Typical moods may be that of "sulking" due to restraint or anger, and being "jumpy" from repressed fear. Of course, it is common for these moods to prevail well into adulthood.

There are differences in intensity of emotions. You will probably recall in your own experience as a nurse that some persons may react rather violently to a situation that, to you, might appear insignificant. This kind of behavior is likely to reflect one's background and past experience with specific kinds of situations.

Emotions are subject to rapid change. A young child is capable of shifting quickly from laughing to crying, or from anger to joy. Although the reason for this is not definitely known, it might be that there is not as much depth of feeling among children as there is among adults. In addition, it could be due to the lack of experience that children have had, as well as their state of intellectual development. We do know that young children have a short attention span, which could cause them to change rapidly from one kind of emotion to another. As we mature into adults, rapid change in emotions is likely to wane.

Depending on the individual, emotions can appear with various degrees of frequency. As individuals grow and mature, they manage to develop the ability to adjust to situations that previously would have caused an emotional reaction. This is, no doubt, due to the acquisition of more experience with various kinds of emotional situations. (This sometimes happens with nurses with long experience; they "mellow" so to speak.) As far as children are concerned, they learn through experience what is socially acceptable and what is socially unacceptable. This is particularly true if a child is reprimanded in some way following a violent emotional reaction. For this reason, a child may try to confront a situation in ways that do not involve an emotional response. You probably know of some adults who tend to react in much the same way.

People differ in their emotional responses. One person confronted with a situation that instills fear may run away from the immediate environment (hit and run driver), while another may try to hide. Different reactions of people to emotional situations are probably due to a host of factors. Included among these may be past experience with a certain kind of emotional situation, willingness of parents and other adults during childhood to help them become more independent, and family relationships in general.

Strength of people's emotions are subject to change. At some age levels certain kinds of emotions may be weak and later become stronger. Conversely, with some children, emotions that were strong tend to decline. For example, young children may be timid among strangers, but later when they see there is nothing to fear, the timidity is likely to diminish. This may be true of some adults who experienced insecurity in childhood.

Emotional Arousals and Reactions

If we are to understand the nature of human emotions, we need to take into account some of those factors of emotional arousal and how people might react to them. Many different kinds of emotional patterns have been identified. For purposes here I have arbitrarily selected for discussion the emotional states of fear, worry, anger, jealousy, and joy.

Fear. The term fear from the Old English *fir* may have been derived originally from the German word *fahr*, meaning danger or peril. In modern times fear is often thought of in terms of anxiety caused by present or impending danger or peril. For example, one authoritative source[2] suggests that fear is generally defined as a more generalized reaction to a vague sense of threat in absence of a specific or realistic dangerous object. However, the terms are often used loosely and almost interchangeably. When fearful or anxious, individuals experience unpleasant changes in overt behavior, subjective feelings (including thoughts), and physiological activity.

Similarly, another source[1] contends that fears differ from anxiety in that the former are negative emotional responses to any specific environmental factor. But fears and anxiety are similar in the feelings they arouse; rapid heartbeat, sweating, quivering, heavy breathing, feeling weak or numb in the limbs, dizziness or faintness, muscular tension, the need to eliminate, and a sense of dread — the "fight or flight" mechanism. Not all people experience all these signs of fear, but most experience some of them.

There are various ways of classifying fears. Spencer Rathus and Jeffrey Nevid[1] use the two broad classifications of *objective* fears and *irrational* fears.

Many objective fears are useful and necessary and it is logical that we be afraid of such things as: (1) touching a hot stove, (2) falling from a high place, (3) running into the street without looking for oncoming vehicles and (4) receiving surgical procedures without benefit of anesthesia. These fears are said to be *rational* and *adaptive*.

Some fears are said to be *irrational* and *maladaptive*. It is an irrational fear when the objective danger is in disproportion to the amount of distress experienced. These kinds of fears are called *phobias* or phobic disorders, among some of which are: (1) fear of high places, though one may be in no objective danger of falling, (2) fear of closed-in, tight places when one is not necessarily in objective danger of being smothered or trapped, (3) fear of receiving injections — not because of the potential minor pain, but because of the "thought" of the procedure (nurses are certainly familiar with this fear in some patients), (4) fear of working with sharp instruments (certainly a detriment for a surgical nurse), (5) fear of the dark, and (6) fear of being alone.

Irrational fears or phobias do not necessarily have to interfere with our lives. It matters little if you are afraid of heights if your life style permits you to avoid high places. However, some irrational fears can be debilitating experiences and interfere greatly with your attempt to lead your daily life. For instance, if one has no tolerance for the sight of blood or being in an environment of medical procedures, one may find his or her health or life endangered if he or she refrains from seeking treatment of an injury or disease. In such a case it would clearly be of benefit to do something about such fears. Of course, the absence of such a fear is a prerequisite for a nurse.

Different people react differently to fears. In my study, ten percent of the nurses said they experienced fear on the job most of the time, 72 percent some of the time and 18 percent said they never had fear on the job. Of the 82 percent experiencing fear most of this was due to the fear of patients failing to recover. Some examples of nurses' fears were:

Fear of getting behind in nursing care.
My fear that I will make an error in judgment.
Fear of permitting physicians to make poor choices in care.
Fear of contracting AIDS.

In some cases particularly among psychiatric nurses, there was fear of mental and physical abuse *from* patients.

Worry. I have already mentioned that this might be considered an imaginary form of fear, and it can be a fear not aroused directly from one's environment. Worry can be aroused by imagining a situation that could possibly arise. Many conscientious nurses worry a great deal about patients only to find such worry unwarranted. This is particularly true of young nurses who are just beginning their careers.

Since worries are likely to be caused by *imaginary* rather than *real* conditions, they are not likely to be found in abundance among very young children. Perhaps the reason for this is that they have not reached a stage of intellectual development where they might imagine certain things that could cause worry. In many adults, worry is a constant problem, and this is true of some nurses I know who will find things to worry about. Controlling worry is a difficult problem for those adults who have problems in adjusting. Eighteen percent of my nurse respondents experienced worry on the job most of the time, and 82 percent experienced worry some of the time.

Anger. One derivation of the word anger is from the Greek word *anchein*, which literally means a strong feeling of displeasure and usually of antagonism. The emotional response to anger tends to occur more frequently than fear. This is probably due to the fact that there are more conditions that incite anger. This has been borne out in some nursing situations with some nurses demonstrating anger toward administration, coworkers, physicians, and patients in this order. In the case of some children, they quickly learn that anger may get attention that otherwise would not be forthcoming; (can you think of any "spoiled" adults who react in this manner?). It is likely that as children get older they may show more anger responses than fear responses because they soon see that there is not as much to fear as they originally thought.

Because of individual differences in people, there is a wide variation in anger responses, and as mentioned previously, these responses are either impulsive or inhibited. It should be recalled that in impulsive responses one manifests an overt action against another person or an object, such as kicking a door. This form of child behavior is also sometimes manifested by some "adults." Twelve percent of the nurses in my survey experienced anger on the job most of the time, 82 percent some of the time, and six percent never experienced anger on the job.

Jealousy. This response usually occurs when one feels a threat of loss of affection. Many psychologists believe that jealousy is closely related to anger. Because of this, a person may build up resentment against another person. Jealousy can be very devastating and every effort should be made to avoid it.

Jealousy is concerned with social interactions that involve persons that one likes. There are various ways in which the individual may respond. These include: (1) being aggressive toward the one he or she is jealous of, or possibly toward others as well, (2) withdrawing from the person whose affections one thinks have been lost, and (3) possible development of an "I don't care" attitude.

In some cases, individuals will not respond in any of the above ways. They might try to excel over the person of whom they are jealous. In other words, they might tend to do things to impress the person whose affections they thought had been lost. My study of nurses showed that 30 percent experienced jealousy on the job some of the time while 70 percent never had this experience on the job.

Joy. This pleasant emotion is one that we strive for because it is so important in maintaining emotional stability. Causes of joy differ from one age level to another, and from one person to another at the same age level. This is to say that what might be a joyful situation for one person might not necessarily be so for another. One nurse may become over-joyed at a patient's recovery while another might view it as just routine.

Joy is expressed in various ways, but the most common are laughing and smiling, the latter being a restrained form of laughter. Some people respond to joy with a state of body relaxation. This is difficult to detect because it has little or no overt manifestation. However, it may be noticed when one compares it with body tension caused by unpleasant emotions. We have all seen the nurse who "heaves a sigh of relief" when learning that a patient is "out of danger." Thirty percent of my nurse respondents experienced joy on the job most of the time, 66 percent some of the time, and only two percent never experienced joy on the job.

Table 2

Percent of Time Nurses Are Involved With Certain Emotions on the Job

Emotion	Most of the Time	Some of the Time	Never
Fear	10%	72%	18%
Worry	18%	82%	0%
Anger	12%	82%	6%
Jealousy	0%	30%	70%
Joy	32%	66%	2%

Factors That Influence Emotionality

If we can consider that one is emotionally fit when the emotions are properly controlled, and he or she is becoming more emotionally stable, then emotional fitness is dependent to a certain extent upon certain factors that influence emotionality. The following is a descriptive list of some of these factors.

Fatigue. There are two types of fatigue, *acute* and *chronic*. Acute fatigue is a natural outcome of sustained or severe exertion. It is due to such physical factors as the accumulation of the by-products of muscular exertion in the blood and to excessive *oxygen debt*—the inability of the body to take in as much oxygen as is being consumed by the muscular work. Psychological consideration may also be important in acute fatigue. That is, an individual who becomes bored with his or her work, and who becomes preoccupied with the discomfort involved, will become fatigued much sooner than if he or she is highly motivated to do the same work, is not bored, and does not think about the discomfort.

Chronic fatigue has reference to fatigue that lasts over extended periods — in contrast with acute fatigue, which tends to be followed by a recovery phase and restoration to normal within a more or less brief period of time. Chronic fatigue may be due to any and a variety of medical conditions (such conditions are the concern of the physician, who should evaluate all cases of chronic fatigue to assure that a disease condition is not responsible). It may also be due to psychological factors such as extreme boredom and/or worry of having to do, over an extended period, what one does not wish to do.

Fatigue tends to predispose people to irritability; consequently, we do things to ward off such as "taking a break" at different times during the day. This may be a "coffee" break or a "snack" break. In this particular regard, some studies show that the hungrier a person is the more prone he or she may be to outbursts of anger.

Inferior Health Status. The same thing holds true here as in the case of fatigue. Temporary poor health, such as colds and the like, tend to make people irritable. In fact, there are studies that show that there are fewer emotional outbursts among healthy individuals than unhealthy individuals.

Intelligence. Studies tend to show that, on the average, persons of low intelligence levels have less emotional control than those with higher levels of intelligence. This may be due to the fact that there may be less frustration if a person is intelligent enough to figure things out. The reverse could also be true because people with high levels of intelligence are better able to perceive things that would be likely to arouse emotions.

Social Environment. In a social environment, where such things as quarreling and unrest exist, a person is predisposed to unpleasant emotional conditions. Likewise work schedules that are too crowded can cause undue emotional excitation among nurses as well as others.

Aspiration Levels. It can make for an emotionally unstable situation if expectations are set beyond one's ability.

All of the above factors can have a negative influence on emotionality. Therefore, insofar as possible efforts should be made by the nurse to eliminate these factors. And those that cannot be completely eliminated should at least be kept under control.

THE EMOTIONALLY HEALTHY NURSE

It seems appropriate to close this chapter by mentioning some of the characteristics of emotionally healthy nurses. As we look at some of the characteristics we must recognize that they are not absolute or static. We are not always happy, and we sometimes find ourselves in situations where we are not overly confident. In fact, sometimes we may feel downright inadequate to solve commonplace problems that occur in our daily lives:

1. Emotionally healthy nurses have achieved basic harmony within themselves and a workable relationship with others, such as physicians and coworkers. They are able to function effectively, and usually happily, even though they are well aware of the limitations and rigors involved in human existence.
2. Emotionally healthy nurses manage to adapt to the demands of environmental conditions with emotional responses that are appropriate in degree and kind to the stimuli and situations and that fall, generally, within the range of what is considered "normal" within various environments.
3. Emotionally healthy nurses face problems directly and seek realistic and plausible solutions to them. They try to free themselves from excessive and unreal anxieties, worries, and fears, even though they are aware that there is much to be concerned with and much to be anxious about in the complex and complicated profession of nursing.
4. Emotionally healthy nurses have developed a guiding philosophy of life and have a set of values that are acceptable to themselves and that are generally in harmony with those values of society that are reasonable and conducive to human happiness.
5. Emotionally healthy nurses accept themselves and are willing to deal with the world as it exists in reality. They accept what cannot be changed at a particular time and place and they build and derive satisfaction within the framework of their own potentialities and those of their environment.
6. Emotionally healthy nurses tend to be happy, and they tend to have an enthusiasm for living. They do not focus their attention exclu-

sively upon what they consider to be their inadequacies, weaknesses, and "bad" qualities. They view those around them in this way, too.

7. Emotionally healthy nurses have a variety of satisfying interests, and they maintain a balance between their work, routine responsibilities, and recreation. They find constructive and satisfying outlets for creative expression in the interests that they undertake.

This list of characteristics of emotionally healthy nurses presents a near-ideal situation and obviously no nurse would operate at these high levels at all times. However, these characteristics might well be considered as suitable guidelines for which nurses might strive to help them deal with and possibly prevent unpleasant emotional stress.

REFERENCES

1. Rathus, Spencer A. and Jeffrey S. Nevid. *Behavior Therapy*, New American Library, 1977.
2. Whitehead, D'ann, Shirley Mariela, and C. Eugene Walker. Use of Systematic Desensitization in the Treatment of Children's Fears. In *Stress in Childhood*, James H. Humphrey (ed.), New York, AMS Press, Inc., 1984.

CHAPTER FIVE

STRESS INDUCING FACTORS IN NURSING AND HOW NURSES TRY TO COPE

MOST OF THE material for the content of this chapter is derived from information received from nurses themselves. That is they were asked to identify their most important cause of stress (stressors) and to indicate the techniques they used to try to cope with such stress.

For the most part, the information obtained from nurses was more or less specific in nature. However, I was also able to discern certain general factors as the data were analyzed. One such generalization involved the area of *self-concerns* and stress, and the following discussion pertains to this factor.

One of the important areas of stress-inducing factors is that which involves personal or self concerns. The following generalized descriptive list takes some of these factors into account with particular reference to nurses.

1. *Self concerns associated with the meeting of personal goals.* Stress is likely to result if goals are set that are too difficult to accomplish. For example, goals may be much higher than a particular environment will permit one to achieve. On the contrary, if we set goals that are too low we can develop the feeling that we are not doing as much as we should. This aspect of stress is also concerned with the fear that some nurses have that they will not reach their goals in their chosen profession. That is, they may believe that their talents could be put to better use in some other career pursuit. Several of the nurses in my survey expressed this point of view and some were in the process of changing careers.

2. *Self concerns which involve self-esteem.* This involves the way a nurse feels about herself, and often self-esteem can be highly related to the

45

fulfillment of certain *ego needs*. Some people may feel that there are not enough opportunities offered in modern society for them to succeed. It bothers some people, too, that their superiors do not praise them for what they consider to be a job well done (I will discuss this later with regard to the nurse-administration relationship). In my interviews with various nurses, many complained that they were rarely complimented when they did a good job but were sometimes criticized for things beyond their control. It is also stressful for some young nurses who feel that they are not advancing as rapidly as they would like in the nursing profession.

Some of the nurses in my survey expressed their feeling about the factor of self-concern and stress with such statements as: "My self-respect and social status are endangered" and "We have unmet self-esteem needs because most people see nurses as custodial caregivers and don't give us credit for the wealth of knowledge we must apply."

3. *Self-concerns related to changing values.* It is frustrating to some nurses if they do not understand the value system imposed on them in a given situation. They may develop the feeling that others are not inclined to place a value on those factors that they feel are important to them personally.

4. *Self concerns that center around social needs.* In some cases nurses may feel that their own social life is neglected because of the demands for "outside" work that is associated with the job. For example, in the profession of nursing, such requirements as changing shifts tend to infringe upon the social life that many nurses feel that they deserve. Some feel, because they need to do outside work to supplement income that not only is their own personal social life being neglected, but that of their family as well. Typical of the expressions of nurses were: "Lack of recognition and social status by patients, physicians, and hospital personnel" and "Irregular hours compared to the rest of society can hamper social status."

5. *Self concerns involving personal competence and ability.* This could be the self concern that frustrates some nurses the most. Certainly, lack of confidence in one's ability can be devastating to the morale of a nurse and some say that they question their own ability when things do not go as well as they expected. Following are statements made by nurses in this regard.

"My fear that I'll make an error in judgment that will result in harm to a patient."

"Fear of not making the right choices in patient care."

"Lack of opportunity to broaden practical skills."
"Inability to give safe nursing care."

CLASSIFICATION OF
STRESS INDUCING FACTORS

As mentioned previously I was able to obtain firsthand from nurses themselves those factors which induced the most stress. This was accomplished by simply requesting that they identify those factors connected with their job that were most stressful for them. Obviously, this resulted in a huge mass of data. It seemed appropriate to sort out the stressors and place them in what appeared to be the most appropriate classifications.

The difficulty encountered in attempting to devise a foolproof system for the classification of nurses' stressors should be obvious. The reason for this, of course, lies in the fact that it is practically impossible to fit a given stressor into one exclusive classification because of the possibilities of overlapping. However, an attempt was made to do so, and it should be made clear that the classification on my part was purely arbitrary. Others might wish to use different classifications than those used here, and in the absence of anything resembling standardization, it would be their prerogative to do so. With this idea in mind, the following classifications of nurses' stressors were finally decided upon:

1. Patients
2. Understaffing
3. Administration
4. Coworkers
5. Time
6. Physicians
7. Compensation
8. Supplies and Equipment

Patients. It is not surprising that patients are a source of stress for nurses (64%). The following wide range of comments made by nurses about patients give some indication of stress that nurses are under when dealing with patients.

- Super-demanding patients
- When a patient is going from bad to worse
- Unstable patients not responding to treatment

Table 3

**Percent of Nurses Who Identified Stressors
in Certain Classifications**

Classification of Stressor	Percent of Nurses Identifying
Patients	64%
Understaffing	50%
Administration	44%
Coworkers	30%
Time	30%
Physicians	24%
Compensation	12%
Supplies and Equipment	10%

- Attempting to help patients when they have no desire to regain health
- Lack of recognition from patients
- Mental stress of dealing with geriatric patients and families
- Lack of respect and compassion from patients
- Concern about unstable patients
- High demands placed on me by patients
- Emotional "neediness" of patients and families
- Too many patients to care for
- Dealing with dying patients
- Dealing with irate family members of patients
- Terminal patient caseload
- Inability to cope with patient demands and their families.
- Interference with patient care by doctors and nursing office
- No one available to help me with patients
- Number of patients requiring total care
- Number of times being interrupted when trying to care for patients
- Being part to the needless suffering of patients as a result of inappropriate use of invasive medical technology
- Severely ill patients requiring a lot of time
- High-risk patients
- No time to communicate with patients
- Very sick patients all the time
- Dealing with critical patients in ICU
- Too many patients leaving no time for meal break and proper patient care

- Trauma patients in OR
- Making important decisions with complex difficult patients

Understaffing. I have arbitrarily used the term understaffing to identify this classification of nursing stressors. It has also been described as:
work pressure,[2] time pressures,[5], work overload,[9] unexpected urgent situations,[8], inadequate staffing,[13] not having enough time and resources
to do the job,[1] and having dual lines of authority to both medical and administrative staff.[4] This classification is a significant source of stress for
nurses and about one half of the nurses in my survey identified it as
such.

In one study[15] workload was significantly related to job dissatisfac-
tion and a reason for many nurses leaving the profession. This was
found in a survey of almost 800 nurses at a large university hospital.
Also understaffing and overwork was the third most frequently cited
source of 52 stressful incidents in a survey of 87 neonatal in-care unit
staff nurses; it accounted for five of the 13 most stressful items.[7] Another
study[14] indicated that 66 percent of nurses reported no leisure time, 33
percent work more than five days in a row, and one-third would prefer
more staff to a 15 percent increase in salary.

Some of the stressors that my nurse respondents cited in this classification follow.

- Short handed and always need more help
- Too large a patient-nurse ratio in the hospital
- People lined up at the door with multiple problems (nurse adminis-
  trator)
- Unstable work environment due to constant change in staff
- Concern of losing staff members due to rapid changes taking place
  in nursing
- Staff shortage from burnout and hospital economics
- Poor staffing and shift schedules
- Making sure all units are adequately staffed (nurse administrator)
- Completion of impossible assigments
- Inefficient staff organization
- Too few nurses for the number of patients
- Too much work to handle
- Lack of coverage overtaxed to point of becoming dangerous for pa-
  tients and nurses
- Unqualified help
- Lack of coverage due to nursing shortage

- Untrained help
- Too many tasks to perform
- Inadequate staffing is the number one stress factor!!!!
- Being overworked

Administration. Forty-four percent of my nurse respondents identified certain aspects of administration as stressful. In one study [6] it was reported that emotional exhaustion in health professions is linked to feelings of lack of control over policies and decisions of doctors and administrators, and fewer opportunities to be creative. In a survey [12] of 232 nurses in a North Carolina hospital it was reported that a supportive organization climate such as open expression of views and joint problem-solving was associated with work group cohesiveness, job satisfaction and less stress. Also supervisor support was shown to be negatively correlated with emotional exhaustion in a survey of 310 Army Medical Center nurses. [2] And finally, lack of staff support was the largest producer of stress among 93 hospice staff (75% of the nurses), a greater stressor than emotional concern for patients and families or managing the disease process. [16]

Some of the typical administration-induced stressors in my survey of nurses included the following.

- Displaced attitudes; that is, paper work over patient care.
- Too little support from hospital administrators
- Administration attitude toward nursing department
- Having little power in terms of administration
- Mismanagement
- Inadequate supervisors
- Added menial tasks not related to skilled care
- Lack of control over working environment
- Paper work when patient's need is great
- Disciplining difficult staff members (nurse administrator)
- Supervisors lack of knowledge of day-to-day workload
- Supervisors who do not know how to manage
- Constant turnover in management
- Most nursing administrators I've encountered are pleasant and average but not the type of bright person I'd like to see influencing the direction of my profession
- Administration expecting too much
- We have a right to expect more loyalty from administrators than they give

- Not respected by administrators for your ability
- Lack of recognition from administration

Coworkers. Thirty percent of the nurses in my survey indicated that they were stressed in some way by their colleagues and coworkers. In this regard it is interesting to note that one study [3] in a survey of 144 nurses at four East Coast city hospitals found that relations with coworkers and supervisors was the largest factor related to job satisfaction, accounting for 24 percent of the variance. Following are some examples of how nurses said they were stressed by coworkers.

- Uncooperative colleagues — late, and not assuming responsibilities
- Ancillary help inconsistent and not dependable
- Incompetence of peers and other employees
- Coworkers who talk nonstop and don't do work
- Personal conflicts with coworkers
- Lazy coworkers
- High demands placed on me by coworkers
- Unqualified or unmotivated assistants
- Lack of motivation of other staff members
- Unprofessional nurses
- Hostile staff
- Coworkers who are not flexible
- When others don't help each other
- Incompetent uncaring coworkers

Time. In most studies on occupational stress well over one-fourth of the respondents cite various factors related to time as serious causes of stress. My study of nurses was no exception with 30 percent citing stressors in this classification. Some responses follow.

- Pressure to deliver more than I am able
- Two or three things that need to be done at once
- Getting behind in nursing care
- Long hours
- Being rushed — too many things to do in a certain time period
- Having to work all shifts and mandatory overtime
- Shift rotation
- Lack of time to do tasks as well as I would like
- Too much to do in too little time
- Not enough time to give safe nursing care
- Irregular hours compared to rest of society

Physicians. It has been reported by one authority[9] that nurses feel "abandoned" by physicians who avoid difficult or dying patients and are not there for emergencies. In addition, in a study[11] of 112 nurses in the Netherlands a clear link was found between problems with physicians and hospital management experienced by nurses, and the nurses' *negative attitudes towards patients*. This is indeed unfortunate because it is extremely important that nurses and physicians work together for the benefit and well-being of their patients. Almost one-fourth of the nurses in my survey indicated that physicians were a cause of stress. Following are some comments that were made in this regard.

- The doctor's anxiety level
- Chauvinistic doctors who think they are God
- Fear of permitting physician to make poor choice in care
- Lack of recognition from physicians
- Irrational and unreasonable MDs
- Doctors' attitudes
- Dealing with old time doctors who are very condescending of my knowledge
- Doctor endangering my self-respect
- When there is a need to call physician at night when there is a condition change in a patient
- Doctors misunderstanding nurse's job
- Demanding attitudes of doctors
- Doctors lack of concern for nurses
- Doctors expecting to have nurses wait on them like maids
- My frustration is compounded by the fact that some unnecessary medical technology is often initiated by a physician to avoid lawsuits down the road
- Dealing with doctors

Compensation. Although low salary is a chief cause of nurses leaving the profession, only 12 percent of my nurse respondents found it to be stressful. Most of these were younger nurses who have been in the profession for a relatively short period of time.

Supplies and Equipment. Ten percent of the nurses in my survey were stressed because of the problem of supplies and equipment. Some of them commented as follows.

- Getting proper supplies and equipment
- Malfunctioning supplies and equipment

- Fighting with auxillary departments like dietary and pharmacy for things you need

HOW NURSES TRY TO COPE

In my survey, nurses were asked to complete two checklists involving things they were presently doing to cope with stress. One such checklist contained what I call "principles of living" to avoid stress. The other checklist involved some of the time-honored stress reduction techniques. These data are reported in the following discussions.

Application of Principles of Living to Avoid Stress

Obviously, there are no resolute standard procedures that are guaranteed to relieve a person entirely from undesirable stress. There are, however, certain general principles of living which may be applied as guidelines to help alleviate stressful conditions.

All life pursuits involve *general* and *specific* factors. In the case of dealing with stress, there are certain general principles that are likely to apply to most individuals. On the other hand, there are certain specific procedures for coping with stress that may be used by an individual in terms of how these procedures might meet his or her particular needs. The present discussion is concerned with some general principles of living to deal with stress that in one way or another can be applied to practically all individuals.

I interpret the term *principle* to mean *guide to action*. Thus, the following principles should be considered as guidelines, but not necessarily in any particular order of importance. Moreover, it should be recognized that each principle is not a separate entity unto itself. This means that all of the principles are in some way interrelated and interdependent upon each other.

PRINCIPLE: Observe Personal Health Practices

Comment: Because of their training and experience, nurses should find this an easy principle to accept, but sometimes it is a difficult one to accomplish. No one is against health, but not everyone abides by those practices that can help maintain a suitable level of health. Nursing, with its imposing work load, may cause nurses to neglect the basic requirements that are essential for the human organism to reach an adequate functional level. Thirty percent of the nurses said they abided by this principle. This leaves almost three-fourths of them who are neglectful of some aspect of health. Chapter Seven is devoted to personal health regimen for nurses to consider.

PRINCIPLE: Engage in a Self-Evaluation of Your Performance

Comment: The practice of constantly taking stock of one's activities can help minimize some of the problems the nurse encounters on the job, or in other aspects of the environment. This can be accomplished in part by taking a little time at the end of each day for an evaluation of the events that occurred during the day, and reactions to those events. Setting aside this time to review performance is important to the achievement of goals. Those who take time to do this will be more likely to identify certain problems over which they have no control, and thus, will try to make an adjustment until such time that a positive change can be effected. The particular time that this task is performed is an individual matter; however, it is not recommended that it be done immediately at the end of the day. A little time should be taken to "unwind" before evaluating actions that took place during the day. Seventy-eight percent of the nurses indicated that they engaged in the practice of self-evaluation.

PRINCIPLE: Try to Recognize Your Own Accomplishments

Comment: A nurse must learn to recognize her own accomplishments and praise herself for them, especially if such praise is not offered by others. This is generally known as "stroking" or "patting one's self on the back." In practicing this procedure a nurse can develop positive attitudes and/or belief systems about her own accomplishments and thus reduce stress. All too often, some nurses "sell themselves short" and do not give themselves credit for the important things that they accomplish. Sixty-two percent of the nurses said they abided by this principle.

PRINCIPLE: Try to Take One Thing at a Time

Comment: I have already mentioned the "time" factor as being stress inducing for some nurses. What we are concerned with here is time budgeting and procrastination. Some nurses are likely to put things off—especially unpleasant things—and as a consequence, frustrations can build up as tasks pile up. There is a need to sort out those tasks in order of importance and attack them one at a time. Proper budgeting of time

Table 4
Percent of Nurses Practicing Certain Principles of Living

Principle	Percent of Nurses Practicing
Talk things over with others	88%
Try to take one thing at a time	80%
Engage in self-evaluation of your performance	78%
Try to recognize your own accomplishments	62%
Try not to take things too seriously	62%
Do things for others	58%
Observe personal health practices	30%

can help alleviate procrastination, which in itself can be a stress inducing factor. Budgeting of time can help eliminate worries of time urgency and the feeling of "too much to do in too short a time." Eighty percent of the nurses practiced this principle.

PRINCIPLE: Try Not to Take Things Too Seriously

Comment: This should not be interpreted to mean that important things like one's job should not be taken seriously. It does mean that there can be a fine line between what is actually serious and what is not. Sometimes when people look back at a particular event, they may wonder how they could have become so excited about it. Those nurses who are able to see the humorous side in their various environments tend to look at a potentially stressful situation more objectively, and this can assist in keeping stress levels low. Sixty-two percent of the nurses said they abide by this principle.

PRINCIPLE: Do Things for Others

Comment: Nurses can sometimes take their mind off their own stressful conditions by offering to do something for other persons. And it can be stated unequivocally that most nurses try to do a great deal for their patients. When individuals are helpful to others, in attempting to relieve them of stress, they in turn will tend to be relieved of stress themselves. Research shows that those persons who volunteer to help others often get as much, if not more, benefit from this practice as those they volunteer to help. Fifty-eight percent of the nurses said that they practice this principle.

PRINCIPLE: Talk Things Over With Others

Comment: Nurses sometimes tend to keep things to themselves, and as a consequence, they may not be aware that others may be disturbed by these same things. Sometimes discussing something with a colleague or with a spouse can help one to see things in a much different light. It is important to keep in mind that such discussions should be positive and objective lest it degenerate into idle gossip. Eighty-eight percent of the nurses said they practiced this principle and in most instances things were talked over with family members.

Specific Stress Reducing Techniques

Nurses were asked to identify those procedures that they found most helpful in relieving them of stress. Some of these techniques were performed as a designated means of reducing stress. Others were engaged in for the sheer enjoyment derived from them; nonetheless, the latter type of activities relieved stress as well. For example, six percent of the nurses reported that *having sex* was found to be most helpful in relieving them of stress. Since this is an activity engaged in by practically all of the adult population, this should not be interpreted to mean that it was used only as a stress reduction technique.

Highlighting some of the items in Table 5, a high percentage (69) *engage in passive recreational activites*. Such activities included reading, listening to music, gardening, and needlework. Sixty-seven percent of the nurses took part in some form of *physical exercise*, including swimming, jogging, walking, tennis, and other net games. It should be mentioned that physical exercise was engaged in on a more or less sporadic and spasmodic basis. Chapter Seven goes into some detail with reference to the benefits of exercise in reducing stress.

Two-fifths of the nurses reduced stress by *inducing the relaxation response* through progressive relaxation, biofeedback, and meditation. These techniques will be discussed in detail in the final chapter. Twenty-four percent resorted to *divine guidance* to reduce stress. Some typical comments of nurses in this regard were as follows.

"I trust in my Lord Jesus Christ."
"God and my family."
"Prayer helps to control stress."
"I find relief from stress when I read the Bible."

Another 24 percent *used alcoholic beverages* and this was done moderately, usually with the traditional cocktail before dinner. *Deep breathing* was popular with 11 percent and some nurses commented on this in the following manner.

"I pause and take a deep breath at work, forget about it, and slow down before going home."

"I take a deep breath and keep going."

Deep breathing will be discussed in Chapter Eight in connection with relaxation. Although only five percent engaged in systematic desensitization as a method of reducing stress, they all found it to be most useful and would highly recommend it to others. This technique is dealt with in detail in Chapter Six as a form of behavior modification.

Table 5
Percent of Nurses Engaging in
Specific Stress Reducing Techniques

Technique	*Percent of Nurses*
Engage in passive recreational activities	69%
Physical exercise	67%
Inducing relaxation response	30%
Divine guidance	24%
Use of alcoholic beverages	24%
Change of scenery (days off, etc.)	13%
Deep breathing	11%
Having sex	6%
Systematic desensitization	5%

REFERENCES

1. Bates, E.M. and B.N. Moore. Stress in Hospital Personnel, *Medical Journal of Australia*, 2, 1975.
2. Constable, J.F. and D.W. Russell. The Effect of Social Support and the Work Environment Upon Burnout of Nurses, *Journal of Human Stress*, 12, 1986.
3. Everly, George S. and R.L. Falcione. Perceived Dimensions of Job Satisfaction for Staff Registered Nurses, *Nursing Research*, 25, 1976.
4. Gray-Toft, P. and J.G. Anderson. Stress Among Hospital Nursing Staff: Its Causes and Effects, *Social Science and Medicine*, 15A, 1981.
5. Ivancevich, J.M. and M.T. Matteson. Nurses and Stress: Time to Examine the Potential Problem, *Supervisor Nurse*, 11, 1980.
6. Jackson, S.E. Organizational Practices for Preventing Burnout, in A.S. Sethi and R.S. Schuler (eds.), *Handbook of Organizational Stress and Coping Strategies*, Cambridge, MA, Ballinger, 1984.
7. Jacobson, S.P. Stressful Situations for Neonatal Intensive Care Nurses, *The*

American Journal of Maternal Child Nursing, 3, 1978.

8. Leppanen, R.A. and M.A. Olkinuora. Psychological Stress Experienced by Health Care Personnel, *Scandinavian Journal of Work, Environment and Health,* 13, 1987.

9. Marshall, J. Stress Amongst Nurses, in C.L. Cooper and J. Marshall (eds.), *White Collar and Professional Stress,* London, Wiley, 1980.

10. Motowildo, S.J., J.S. Packard, and M.R. Manning. Occupational Stress: Its Causes and Consequences for Job Performance, *Journal of Applied Psychology,* 71, 1986.

11. Nievard, A.C. Communication Climate and Patient Care: Causes and Effects of Nurses' Attitudes to Patients, *Social Science and Medicine,* 24, 1987.

12. Revicki, D.A. and H.J. May. Organizational Characteristics, Occupational Stress and Mental Health in Nurses. Paper presented at the American Public Health Association, Anaheim, CA, November, 1984.

13. Scully, R. Stress in the Nurse, *American Journal of Nursing,* 80, 1980.

14. Sexton, P. *The New Nightingales,* New York, Enquiry Press, 1982.

15. Weisman, C.S., C.S. Alexander, and G.A. Chase. Determinants of Hospital Staff Nurse Turnover, *Medical Care,* 19, 1981.

16. Yancik, R. Sources of Work Stress for Hospice Staff, *Journal of Psychological Oncology,* 2, 1984.

CHAPTER SIX

SELF-MODIFICATION OF BEHAVIOR AS A STRESS REDUCING TECHNIQUE FOR NURSES

FOR PURPOSES of this discussion I will consider *behavior* as anything that the organism does as a result of some sort of stimulation. I will consider the term *modification* to mean a change in the organism caused by environmental factors. Thus, when the two terms are used together—behavior modification—they are interpreted to mean some sort of change in the way a person has ordinarily reacted to a given stimulus.

It is not uncommon for some individuals to display behavior that directly or indirectly causes stress arousal, either for themselves and/or for the person(s) toward whom the behavioral action is directed. It is the function of this chapter to provide information that will assist nurses to modify behavior for the purpose of correcting or at least improving upon this condition.

In recent years, behavior modification has become so broad in scope that it is used in many frames of reference. I would like to emphasize at this point that, for my purposes, I am not considering it as a variety of psychological and/or psychiatric techniques (therapist-client relations) for altering behavior. On the contrary, my recommendations for the use of modification of behavior are confined to its possibilities as a means for nurses to reduce certain stress-connected factors involved in their working environment. This is to say that if a nurse manifests a behavior that provokes a stressful situation, if she can change this behavior, it could be possible to eliminate, or at least minimize the stressful condition. For example, let us say that if a nurse constantly uses what others consider to be unwarranted criticism, this can create a problem in social relationships and thus a stressful atmosphere.

In general, the practice of behavior modification involves external assistance as in the case of a nurse trying to effect a change in a patient. The major concern here is in the direction of *self*-modification with the nurse attempting to improve her own behavior. This assumes that, generally speaking, nurses can help themselves develop the ability to increase desirable or appropriate behavior and to decrease undesirable or inappropriate behavior. Of course, this involves self-control, which can be described as manipulation of environmental events that influence one's own behavior for the purpose of changing the behavior. Self-control can eventually lead to behavioral self-management, which can be considered as the learning and practice of new habits. Satisfactory self-control and successful self-management are obviously contingent upon some sort of understanding of self, and this is the subject of the ensuing discussion.

TOWARD AN UNDERSTANDING OF SELF

In order to put an understanding of self in its proper perspective, consideration needs to be given to the basic aspect of *self-structure* and *self-concept*. Hugh Perkins,[3] one of my former associates and a leading learning theorist suggests that self-structure is the framework of a particular individual's complex of motives, perceptions, cognitions, feelings, and values — the product of developmental processes. Self-structure is revealed in behavior. One reveals in behavior the knowledge, skills, and interests that have been acquired, the goals being sought, the beliefs, values, and attitudes adopted, the roles learned, and the self-concept that has been formed. Thus, self-concept is an aspect of self-structure.

It is also suggested that among the most relevant and significant perceptions that an individual acquires are those of himself or herself in various life situations; and further, that basically, the self-concept is made up of a large number of *percepts*, each of which contains one or more qualities that one ascribes to himself or herself. To be more specific, *self-percept* pertains to sense impressions of a trait ascribed to, while *self-concept* consists of the totality of one's self-percepts organized in some sort of order.

The frame of reference of self-concept with which I am concerned involves the *total personality* concept. A great deal of clinical and experimental evidence indicates that a human being must be considered as a whole and not a collection of parts, and thus, is a total personality.

A question to raise is, "What comprises the total personality?" Anyone who has difficulty formulating views with regard to what the human personality actually consists of can take courage in the knowledge that many experts who spend their time studying it are not always in complete agreement as to what it is or how it operates. However, if one were to analyze the literature on the subject, it would be found generally, that the total personality consists of the sum of all the *physical, social, emotional,* and *intellectual* aspects of any individual. This can also be expressed in terms of the physical self, social self, emotional self, and intellectual self with everyone manifesting certain kinds of physical behavior, social behavior, emotional behavior, and intellectual behavior. (Although this discussion deals with self-concept in a general way, as you read on, you will no doubt want to visualize the way in which "your own self" corresponds to the general pattern. The importance of this approach is seen when you as an individual make an effort in the direction of self modification of behavior.)

The total personality is one thing comprising the above major aspects. All of these components are highly interrelated and interdependent. All are important to the balance and health of the personality because only in terms of their health can the personality as a whole maintain a completely healthy state. The condition of any one aspect affects each other aspect to a degree, and hence, the personality as a whole.

When a nervous person stutters or becomes nauseated, a mental state is not necessarily causing a physical symptom. On the contrary, a pressure imposed upon the organism causes a series of reactions, which include thought, verbalization, digestive processes, and muscular function. Mind does not always cause the body to become upset; the total organism is upset by a situation, and reflects its upset in several ways, including disturbance in thought, feeling, and bodily processes. The whole individual responds in interaction with the social and physical environment, and as the individual is affected by the environment, he or she in turn has an effect upon it.

Because of long tradition during which physical development *or* intellectual development, rather than physical *and* intellectual development, has been glorified, we oftentimes are still accustomed to dividing the two in our thinking. The result may be that we sometimes pull human beings apart with this kind of thinking.

Traditional attitudes, which tended to separate mind and body, perhaps, led to unbalanced development of an individual with respect to mind and body and/or social adjustment. To understand better the concept of total personality the human organism is represented in the schematic diagram in Figure 1.

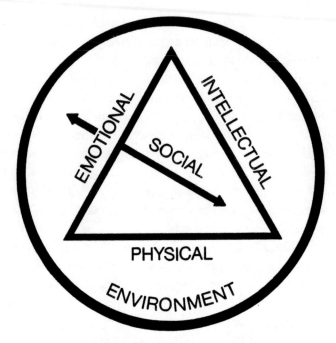

Figure 1. Schematic diagram of "total personality."

The circle is the total environment of the individual, which circumscribes and confines all aspects of the total personality. The triangle with its three sides—physical, emotional, and intellectual aspects of the total personality—form a single figure. An arrow extending from the center of the triangle upward through one of the sides, is designated *social* to represent the interpersonal relationships within the field of the individual and the environment. The arrow is pointed at both ends to suggest a two-way process; the individual is affected by others and he or she in turn has some effect upon them. The triangle is dependent upon a balance of all its parts, and if one part of the triangle is changed, the entire triangle is reshaped. It is interesting to draw diagrams in which one after the other of the sides is shortened—as in one kind or another of personality limitations—and see how this affects the triangle. You may also find it interesting to make personal applications such as the following: What happens to my intellectual peformance when I am worried or have a stomachache? What changes occur in my body when I feel frightened, embarrassed, or angered?

It is interesting in modern times, when great emphasis is placed upon social adjustment, that perhaps a major problem involves faulty interpersonal relationships. For this reason, it is important to make special note of the interaction between the individual and the environment. The quality of the individual's interpersonal relationships affects all other aspects of his or her personality. How well do you drive a car when someone is shouting at you? How well can you concentrate when you think someone is talking about you? These are social circumstances that affect the physical, social, emotional, and intellectual aspects of personality.

All of these things, then, are the basis of total personality — a complex balance of psychological and social considerations that prepares the individual for the fullest, most socially valuable, productive, and adventuresome living. A large portion of the responsibility falls to the individual to make those kinds of modifications in personal behavior that will in one way or another add to the quality of living and help in the prevention of undesirable stress.

PROCESSES OF BEHAVIOR ADJUSTMENT

The term *adjustment* can be described as the process of finding and adopting modes of behavior suitable to the environment or to changes in the environment. In fact, at least one authoritative source[1] has described stress as environmental conditions that require behavioral adjustment.

Daily living involves a continuous sequence of experiences characterized by the necessity for the human organism to adjust. Consequently, it may be said that "normal" behavior is the result of successful adjustment, and abnormal behavior results from unsuccessful adjustment. The degree of adjustment that one achieves depends upon how adequately he or she is able to satisfy basic needs and fulfill desires within the framework of the environment and the pattern or ways dictated by society.

As previously mentioned, we tend to think of stress as any factor acting internally or externally that renders adaptation difficult, and induces increased effort on the part of the person to maintain a state of equilibrium within himself or herself and with the external environment. The following points were made previously and are repeated here for purposes of continuity. When stress is induced as a result of the individual's not being able to meet needs (basic demands) and satisfy desires (wants or wishes), *frustration* or *conflict* results. Frustration occurs when a need is not met; and conflict results when choices must be made between nearly equally attractive alternatives or when basic emotional forces oppose one another. In the emotionally healthy person, the degree of frustration is ordinarily in proportion to the intensity of the need or desire. That is, he or she will objectively observe and evaluate the situation to ascertain if a solution is possible, and if so, what solution would best enable him or her to achieve the fulfillment of needs or desires. However, every person has a *zone of tolerance* or limits for physical, physiological, and psychological stress within which he or she normally operates. If the stress becomes considerably greater than the tolerance level, or if the individual has not learned to cope with problems and objectively and intelligently solve them, some degree of maladjustment can possibly result.

SOME GENERAL PROCEDURES FOR SELF-MODIFICATION OF BEHAVIOR

Over the last several years a voluminous amount of literature has been published in the general area of behavior modification. Some of this has been directed to school administrators, teachers, counselors as well as nursing supervisors for the purpose of utilizing the procedure to produce behavior change in others. As mentioned before, I am concerned here with *self*-modification of behavior and literature in this specific area is becoming more abundant.

Although self-modification of behavior is considered to be a relatively recent innovation, one report suggests that it was used in the early history of our country by Benjamin Franklin.[2] He is said to have used it to improve upon such virtues as temperance and frugality. He kept a record of the errors he thought he made each day in each of over a dozen virtues. At the end of the day, he would consult the information to get feedback to help him identify those virtues he may have been violating. Of course, in modern times our approach to self-modification of behavior is much more sophisticated than that of Franklin, and improvement is constantly being made.

Whether one is attempting to modify behavior of another (nursing supervisor with a student nurse) or trying to modify his or her own behavior, the general procedure of application is essentially the same. There are certain sequential steps to be taken that involve the following: (1) identification and description of one's behaviors, (2) counting behaviors, (3) attempting to effect a change in behaviors, and (4) evaluating the procedures used to change behaviors. The following discussion will take into account some of the important features involved in these various steps.

Identifying Behaviors

The first step in the process is concerned with identification of a behavior that one wishes to modify. This process is also referred to as *pinpointing, targeting,* or *specifying* a behavior. Essentially this involves trying to define a particular behavior (target) that one wishes to change. This is not always an easy matter because sometimes a person may manifest a behavior that is annoying to others, but he or she may be completely unaware of it.

When a person is able to identify a particular behavior and admit that such a behavior may be interfering with social relationships, a strong beginning can be made in the direction of behavioral change. In other words, recognizing that one has a problem is the first prerequisite to solving it.

In many instances, the identification of a behavior emerges when one is dissatisfied with what one may be doing. For example, a person may be performing a behavior he or she does not want to perform, or not be performing a behavior he or she wants to perform.

Counting Behaviors

The second step in self-modification of behavior is concerned with actually counting how often a target behavior occurs. This means that one obtains a frequency count of the behavior to be improved. If this step is not taken, it is difficult to learn the extent to which the behavior is being performed. Sometimes, simply counting a behavior will tend to improve it because the person is becoming involved in self-awareness of the behavior. This is to say that counting a behavior calls one's attention to it and how often it is occurring.

In addition to determining the frequency of a behavior, another aspect of this step is what is sometimes called the *ABC Factor* in the behavior modification approach. That is *A*ntecedent of the behavior, the *B*ehavior itself, and the *C*onsequence of the behavior. *Antecedent* is concerned with any event that preceded the behavior and *consequence* is what happens as a result of the behavior.

Obviously, it is most important that a person develop an awareness of antecedents and consequences of behaviors. The main reason for this is that an antecedent gets a behavior started and a given behavior can result in an unsatisfactory consequence.

Attempting to analyze an antecedent becomes important in terms of a manifested behavior. That is, why did the antecedent occur in the first place?

The information derived from step two in self-modification of behavior is usually designated as *baseline data*. If the information is valid and the behavior frequency is accurate, the person has a base from which to operate. This means that one should be in a position to see if attempts at improving a given behavior — step three, *changing behavior* is meeting with satisfactory results.

Changing Behaviors

Any effort to change a behavior that has been identified, described, counted, and recorded is referred to as a *plan of intervention*. That is, the person intervenes with one or more procedures designed to modify the inappropriate behavior. Any plan to replace an inappropriate behavior with an appropriate one involves some sort of reinforcement procedure. Generally speaking, *self*-reinforcement is concerned with changing behavior through *self*-produced consequences, and these consequences may be overt or covert. Examples are statements to oneself or the acquisition of an item as a reward for one's efforts.

Evaluating the Plan of Intervention

The final step in self-modification of behavior is concerned with how well the plan of intervention is succeeding; that is, the extent to which the changes in behavior are achieving desired results. This process requires the development of valid evaluative criteria. These criteria can be broad in scope, and thus apply to any problem of self-modification of behavior, or they can be more specific and be applied to a particular case. Some examples of general criteria might include the following:

1. In general, was there an increase in appropriate behavior and/or a decrease in inappropriate behavior?
2. What were the behaviors that achieved the most satisfactory results?
3. What forms of reinforcement appeared to be most successful?

Whatever way one decides to evaluate the plan of intervention, there is still another decision to be made. This also concerns the extent to which the plan has achieved success. If it has met with complete and unequivocal success, it can then perhaps be terminated. Or, if it succeeds only when the behavior change is still being practiced, there may need to maintain the procedure. Perhaps the ultimate goal should be to modify behavior to the extent that the problem would be completely eliminated. This can be accomplished if one conscientiously and systematically carries out the general procedures outlined above. Experiences have shown that nurses can modify their own behavior not only to correct stress arousal but to avoid it as well.

SYSTEMATIC SELF-DESENSITIZATION

A form of behavior modification known as systematic desensitization can be described as the process of systematically lessening a specific learned fear in an individual. It is purported to provide one means of controlling anxiety. If one can accomplish this, it becomes an extremely important factor in reducing stress. The reason for this is that the individual becomes more able to control his or her fears and anxieties, rather than being controlled by them. From the point of view of a clinical psychotherapeutic procedure, systematic desensitization consists of presenting to the imagination of the deeply relaxed person the feeblest item in a list of anxiety-evoking stimuli repeatedly, until no more anxiety is evoked. The next item on the list is presented, and so on, until eventually, even the strongest of the anxiety evoking stimuli fails to evoke any stir of anxiety in the person. It is the purpose here to provide information to help the nurse understand the process of this technique and at the same time give consideration to self-administration for the ultimate purpose of reducing stress.

Originally, the focus of systematic desensitization was primarily upon counselor-client, therapist-patient, or teacher-student relationships, and it was perhaps one of the most widely used behavior therapy techniques. In recent years, systematic desensitization has gained great favor as a *self*-administered technique. Although the value of it as a means of lessening stress-provoking situations has not been completely established by behavioral scientists, some of the research findings are indeed encouraging. For example, studies have shown that systematic self-desensitization can be very effective in overcoming severe public speaking anxiety, test anxiety, and a host of other stress-invoking stimuli.

It has been suggested by one authoritative source[5] that systematic self-desensitization efforts are not likely to be harmful, even if they fail. However, self-desensitization should be approached as an experimental procedure and it should be discontinued if the course of anxiety-reduction is not relatively smooth, and it should be discontinued immediately if any increase in anxiety is experienced.

Various behavioral therapists and clinical psychologists have set forth models for the practice of systematic self-desensitization. One impressive model which seems to have universal applicability is one suggested by one of my collaborators in other stress projects, C. Eugene Walker, chief of pediatric psychology at the University of Oklahoma Medical School.[4]

The subject of systematic desensitization is introduced with the notion that many anxieties that people experience are due to what are termed *conditional reactions*. These conditioned reactions are identified as stimuli that occur together in our experience and become associated with each other so that we respond to them in the same way, or in a highly similar way, when they occur again. This is to say that if we are made anxious in the presence of certain stimuli these same stimuli will make us anxious later when they occur, even if the situation in reality no longer poses an actual threat. An example is a person who may have had a number of experiences as a child in which a person in authority, such as a school principal, policeman, or guard frightened him or her and was perhaps punished in some way. Such a person's reactions as an adult to one in authority may produce considerably more anxiety than the situation really justifies. This is because of previous conditioning of strong anxiety to an authority figure.

Many of our emotions seem to be based on such conditioned reactions. And, these reactions are somewhat similar to reflexes, but they are learned rather than inherited (the reader is asked to refer back to the discussion of learned and unlearned tensions in Chapter Two). Their automatic or "reflexive" character, however, explains why it is difficult to discuss things rationally with someone who is emotionally involved in a situation. Such a person is responding more with conditioned reactions to the present stimuli than relating to the actual realities of the situation.

The recommendation for overcoming anxieties in the form of conditioned reactions is the use of systematic self-desensitization and a highly persuasive case can be made for its effectiveness—provided it is done properly.

After a particular problem has been identified, the process consists of three sequential steps: (1) developing a hierarchy of anxiety-evoking stimuli, (2) complete relaxation, and (3) desensitization sessions. Using the previously mentioned authority figure example, let me make application of this to a nurse who has difficulty with this problem where relationship with a given physician is concerned. Incidentally, my surveys show that it is not uncommon for some nurses to have what they designate as a "fear of the physician" without being able to identify specific reasons for it. In fact, some nurses feel some degree of subserviency to physicians. In many cases this condition is not warranted because nurses should be considered as allies to physicians and not merely as "bed makers" and "tray handlers."

The first step is to take several index cards, writing a different situation or experience on each card that makes for anxiety concerning the problem. The cards are then stacked in order with the one causing the least anxiety on the top and the one causing the greatest anxiety at the bottom. This is the hierarchy of anxiety-evoking stimuli and might resemble the following:

1. Entering the hospital parking lot and seeing the physician's car.
2. Greeting other nurses and discussing the physician.
3. Greeting a nurse who mentions her association with the physician.
4. Conferring with another nurse about her relationship with the physician.
5. Walking by physician's office when the door is closed.
6. Walking by physician's office when the door is open (no verbalization or eye contact).
7. Walking by physician's office when door is open using eye contact and nodding.
8. Arranging meeting with physician's secretary.
9. Talking with physician's secretary about the physician.
10. Prearranged meeting with physician with secretary present.
11. Prearranged meeting with physician with only self present.
12. Other meetings with the physician with only self present.

Another possible stress-inducing situation that concerns some nurses is that of making a report in front of a group. A hierarchy that one nurse used for self-desensitization follows:

1. Reading an article about giving reports.
2. Reading report alone.
3. Reading report in front of a mirror.
4. Reading report into tape recorder and playing back.
5. Reading report to a friend.
6. Reading report to a friend with one other present.
7. Reading report with three others present.
8. Reading report to two or three where there is a large gathering, such as the lunchroom.

9. Entering the room where the report is to be given.
10. Member of audience where reports are given.
11. Giving report to entire group.

Of course the reader must understand that the above hierarchies of anxiety-evoking stimuli are general in nature and each individual would make out his or her list in more specific detail and pertaining to more specific anxieties.

The second step is to try to develop a condition of complete relaxation (the reader is referred to the final chapter for information about various relaxation procedures).

After the nurse is completely relaxed, the next step is the beginning of systematic self-desensitization. This is done as follows: Look at the top card of the pile—the one that is the least anxiety provoking. Close the eyes, and using the imagination, visualize as vividly as possible the situation described on it. That is, you imagine the situation occurring and that you are actually there. At this point, if some anxiety is experienced, the imaginary scene should cease immediately and you should go back to relaxing. After complete relaxation is again obtained, you are ready to proceed. This procedure is continued until the scene can be imagined without anxiety. This may take only one or two times, or it could take 15 to 20 times, but it should be repeated until no anxiety is felt. The entire procedure is continued until you have gone through all the cards.

It is recommended that you work on the scenes in this manner for approximately one-half hour at a time. It can be done daily, every other day, or a couple of times a week, depending upon the amount of time you are willing or able to spend, and how quickly you want to conquer the anxiety. It appears to be a good practice to overlap one or two items from one session to another; that is, beginning a session by repeating an item or two from the previous session that were imagined without anxiety.

One variation of the above procedure is to tape record a description of each scene in advance. You then relax and listen to the tape. If anxiety appears, the recorder is turned off and you go back to relaxing. When relaxation is again accomplished proceed as before. A value of using the tape recorder is that there is likely to be better pronunciation, enunciation, and intonation of words. In addition, it may be easier for you to concentrate since you have your own auditory input on tape and do not have the additional task of verbalizing and trying to concentrate on the scene at the same time. If desired, the sequence of relaxation procedures can be taped as well.

After you have been desensitized, you can review in your own mind the preferred action to take in the situation that caused anxiety. Plans can then be made to do the right thing the next time the situation occurs.

Obviously, the success you experience with this procedure will depend largely upon the extent to which you are willing to make the painstaking effort involved in the approach. I have proposed this procedure to many nurses, and those who have tried it have been so delighted by its effects that they have deliberately sought out situations that previously had caused them great anxiety, frustration, and failure. This is certainly a true test of faith in the approach.

REFERENCES

1. Benson, Herbert. *The Relaxation Response,* New York, William Morrow and Company, Inc., 1975.
2. Knapp, T.J. and S.A. Shodahl. "Ben Franklin as a Behavior Modifier: A Note," *Behavior Therapy,* 5, 1974.
3. Perkins, Hugh. *Human Development and Learning,* 2nd ed., Belmont, CA, Wadsworth Publishing Company, 1974.
4. Walker, C. Eugene. *Learn to Relax, 13 Ways to Reduce Tension,* Englewood Cliffs, NJ, Prentice-Hall, 1975.
5. Watson, David L. and Roland G. Tharp. *Self-Directed Behavior: Self Modification for Personal Adjustment,* Belmont, CA, Wadsworth Publishing Company, 1972.

CHAPTER SEVEN

STRESS MANAGEMENT PERSONAL HEALTH REGIMEN FOR NURSES

HAVING TAUGHT courses for nurses at a large university as well as an army hospital, I am well aware of their educational background in areas related to health. However, such a background does not necessarily guarantee that a nurse will have a complete perception of health as it is concerned with stress.

Although a fair percentage of nurses in my survey said they engaged in personal health practices, at the same time many indicated that they did not do as well as they should in this area. Some admitted to neglecting sleep and rest and others said that their eating habits could be improved. Indeed, basic to the control and reduction of stress is the attention nurses pay to their own personal health.

There appears to be two general factors to consider with regard to stress and health. First, objective evidence continues to accumulate to support the idea that prolonged stressful conditions can be most detrimental to the health of some individuals. And second, along with new and modern techniques of relieving stress, are many traditional health practices that long have enabled people to gain greater control over the tempo of their lives and reduce the disabling effects of stressful living. It is the primary function of this chapter to deal with the second factor in the hope that the discussions will have a positive impact upon eliminating, or at least minimizing the conditions concerned with the first factor. To this end, subsequent major discussions in the chapter will deal with what I call the *fitness triangle:* (1) nutrition and diet, (2) sleep and rest, and (3) physical activity and exercise. However, before getting into specific discussions on these various areas, it seems appropriate to give some consideration to the general area of health.

73

THE MEANING OF HEALTH

The precise meaning that one associates with the term *health* depends in a large measure upon the particular frame of reference in which it is used. In recent years it was a relatively common practice to think of health in terms of the condition of the living organism that functioned normally. This idea about health is one that is still accepted by many people. In subscribing to this particular concept, these individuals tend to think of health predominantly as a state in which there is absence of pain or symptoms related to a poorly functioning organism. When thought of only in this manner, health is considered primarily in terms of a state in which there is absence of disease.

In modern times, health is being considered more and more in terms of *well-being*, which is perhaps our most important human value. In considering health from a point of view of well-being, the ideal state of health would be one in which all of the various parts of the human organism function at an optimal level at all times. Although it is very unlikely that the human organism will ever achieve the ideal state suggested here, such a level is ordinarily used as a standard for diagnosing or appraising the human health status.

The old meaning of health that considered it primarily only in terms of absence of disease tended to place it in a negative sense. The more modern concept places more positive emphasis on the term. This is to say that the meaning of health is interpreted as a level of well-being as well. It seems logical to assume that modern society's goal should be directed toward achieving the highest level of well-being for all of its citizens.

HEALTH KNOWLEDGE, ATTITUDES, AND PRACTICE

Any discussion of health should consider the three important aspects of health knowledge, health attitudes, and health practice. Each of these dimensions will be dealt with separately, but it appears important at the outset to consider them together for the purpose of a better understanding of how they are related.

In order to benefit most from health learning experiences, it is most important that these experiences develop into desirable health practices. Thus, the ultimate goal should be in the direction of a kind of behavior that will be likely to insure optimum present and future health for the individual. However, before the most desirable and worthwhile health practices can be achieved, there is a need for a certain amount of desirable health knowledge, along with a proper attitude, in making appropriate application of the knowledge to health practice.

Although it is obvious that *to know* is not necessarily *to do;* nevertheless, that which is done wisely will depend in a large measure upon the kind and amount of knowledge one has acquired. In the accumulation of health knowledge, one will need to understand why it is beneficial to follow a certain practice. When one knows why, it is perhaps more likely that a desirable attitude toward certain health practices will be developed. If a nurse has a sufficient amount of desirable health knowledge developed through valid health concepts, and also has a proper attitude, he or she will be more apt to apply the knowledge in health behavior. Moreover, he or she should be in a better position to exercise good judgment and make wise decisions in matters pertaining to health if the right kind and amount of health knowledge has been obtained.

Health Knowledge

Knowledge about health is acquired in a variety of different ways. Some of it is the product of tradition and, as such, oftentimes is nothing more than folklore. Certain popular notions about health-related matters that have long since been dispelled by the scientific community, are still held by many people who have not, for some reason or other, benefitted from modern health knowledge.

Other kinds of health knowledge of sorts are derived in our modern society from the constant bombardment of the eyes and ears of people through mass communication media, such as television and radio. Although some of this information may be valid from a health point of view, we should be alert to the possibility that the primary purpose of many kinds of advertising is to sell a product that proclaims results that are not always likely to be attainable.

Another source of health knowledge is the home. In fact, most of our important health learnings get their start in the home. Parents are our first teachers and, for better or for worse, what we learn from them, mostly without our being aware that we are learning it, tends to remain with us. A good home should contribute much to the health knowledge of its children simply by providing good meals and a friendly, well-regulated, but pleasant and recreationally-challenging environment in which to grow. Children from such homes ordinarily do not have to un-learn a lot of faulty ideas and unwholesome attitudes when they are in the next great potential source of health knowledge—the schools. It should be borne in mind that many children who grow up in homes in the inner city and some remote parts of the country do not benefit from good home experiences and thus, their first source of health knowledge is the school.

The scope of knowledge that one might obtain about matters related to health is almost endless, and obviously, it would be impossible to learn all there is to know about it. However, there are certain basic con-cepts about health that should be developed by individuals at all age levels. Generally speaking, the individual should acquire knowledge pertaining to the direct basic needs of the organism, and, in addition, knowledge regarding the human organism as it functions in its environ-ment.

Health Attitudes

Any discussion of attitudes requires an identification of the meaning of the term. Although it is recognized that different people will attach different meanings to the term attitude, for purposes here I would like to think of attitude as being associated with *feelings*. We hear such expres-sions as, "How do you *feel* about it?" In a sense this implies, "What is your *attitude* toward it?" Therefore, theoretically, at least, attitude could be considered a factor in the determination of action because of this feel-ing about something. For example, knowledge alone that physical exer-cise is beneficial will not necessarily lead to regular exercising, but a strong feeling or attitude might be a determining factor that leads one to exercise regularly.

It should be mentioned at this point that, contrary to abundant em-pirical thought, there is little or no objective evidence to support un-equivocally the contention that attitude has a positive direct influence on behavior. One of the difficulties in studying this phenomenon scientifi-cally lies in the questionable validity of instruments used to measure at-titudes. Moreover, there is little consistent agreement with regard to the meaning of attitudes. Thus, the position taken here is one of theoretical postulation based upon logical assumption.

As far as health attitudes are concerned, they could well be consid-ered a gap that can possibly exist between health knowledge and health practice, and this gap needs to be bridged if effective health behavior is to result from acquiring valid health knowledge. Let us consider, as an example, a person who has acquired some knowledge regarding the degree to which cigarette smoking can be harmful to health. Perhaps this person will have some sort of underlying feeling toward such knowledge. He or she may choose to disregard it because friends have also assumed such an attitude toward it. Or, it may be felt that the evidence is convincing enough to believe that cigarette smoking is something that he or she can get along without. In either case an attitude has developed toward the practice of cigarette smoking, and it is likely that one may react in accordance with this feeling. It should also be mentioned that one may not necessarily react in accordance with true feelings because it may be considered fashionable to smoke cigarettes so as not to lose status with friends who do. Whatever way one chooses to react will be tempered at least to an extent by the consequences associated with the knowledge acquired about cigarette smoking.

Obviously, it would be hoped that the accumulation of health knowledge would be accompanied by a positive attitude, and that this attitude would result in desirable action. It is possible that only in terms of such a positive attitude are desirable health practices, and thus, a better way of living likely to result.

Health Practice

It is a well-known fact that all people do not capitalize on the knowledge they have acquired. Perhaps many are apt to act only on impulse; actions of others are influenced to an extent by their friends. However, in a matter as important as one's health, it appears that a reasonable course to follow would be one in which the individual weighs the facts and scientific evidence before acting.

Perhaps we might look at health practices that are desirable and those that are undesirable, or, in other words, those health practices that will result in pleasantness or unpleasantness. If we weigh knowledge in these terms, perhaps we can appreciate better the possible consequence of certain health practices.

Altering behavior is not always an easy matter; however, it is hoped that most persons will want to make a positive modification of their own health behavior after acquiring desirable health knowledge and forming favorable attitudes. In the final analysis, the individual will make the decisions regarding his or her own health practices. In young children, perhaps these health practices can be forced, although this notion is impractical if we expect the best learning to take place; and forcing health practices upon children as they grow older not only appears impractical, but in many cases, unwarranted as well. It is very likely that this same philosophy can be applied to adults.

As far as personal health is concerned, it perhaps becomes a matter of how much risk one is willing to take, and health practices are likely to be based on this factor. By way of illustration I will refer again to cigarette smoking and health. To my knowledge, it has never been demonstrated scientifically that cigarette smoking is in any way beneficial to the physical health of the human organism. On the contrary, there has been a great deal of information accepted as evidence from a medical point of view that indicates that smoking can contribute to certain types of serious diseases. Yet, untold numbers of individuals are willing to assume a dangerous risk in defiance of such evidence. After a person has learned about some aspect of health, he or she is left with an element of choice. It is hoped a course of action would be chosen that would involve a minimum of risk.

NUTRITION

Nutrition can be descibed as the sum of the processes by which a person takes in and utilizes food substances; that is, the nourishment of the body by food. These processes consist of (1) ingestion, (2) digestion, (3) absorption, and (4) assimilation.

Ingestion derives from the Latin word *ingestus* meaning to take in, and in this context it means taking in food, or the act of eating. The process of *digestion* involves the breaking down or conversion of food into substances that can be *absorbed* through the lining of the intestinal tract and into the blood and used by the body. *Assimilation* is concerned with the incorporation or conversion of nutrients into *protoplasm* which is the essential material making up living cells.

Essential Nutrients and Their Function in the Body

The body needs many nutrients or foods to keep it functioning properly. These nutrients fall into the broad groups of proteins, carbohydrates, fats, vitamins, and minerals. (Although water is not a nutrient in the strictest sense of the word, it must be included, for nutrition cannot take place without it.)

Three major functions of nutrients are: (1) building and repair of all body tissues, (2) regulation of all body functions, and (3) providing fuel for the body's energy needs. Although all of the nutrients can do their best work when they are in combination with other nutrients, each still has its own vital role to play.

Protein

Protein is the protoplasmic matter from which all living animal cells and tissues are formed. It is the source of nitrogen, and it is from nitrogen that the building blocks of protein are formed. These basic substances are called *amino acids*, and they are to be found in plant and animal food sources.

The amino acids are acted upon and released during the digestive process, absorbed, and then rebuilt into new protein forms. For example, when you eat a protein food, such as meat, the digestive process promptly breaks it down into various amino acids. The body chemistry then goes to work to reassemble these amino acids into a new protein form. Some of the combinations are used to make cells for different tissues, such as muscle, blood, bone, and the soft tissues of the vital organs. Other amino acid combinations form the various hormones for the endocrine system, and still others are utilized to form enzymes. Enzymes are internal secretions necessary for the proper functioning of the blood, stomach, and other organs of the body. They are highly specialized and are responsible for such varied functions as aiding in the clotting of the blood and turning starches into sugar. It has been found recently that a repeated exposure to a given food may wear out the enzyme system needed to digest that food thus, possibly predisposing one to a food allergy.[8] This could be a consideration in the use of "left over" food.

As an individual ages, there is a gradual loss of total body protein that is largely related to a diminution in the size of the body's muscles. With older individuals there is frequently superimposed infections, reduced gastrointestinal tract functioning and other stress-related metabolic changes which reduce the efficiency of dietary protein intake.

Carbohydrates

Carbohydrates are the fuel foods which provide us with most of the energy to carry on bodily activities, including those associated with basic metabolic processes. All foods provide energy to some extent, but the starches and sugars are the most economical and most easily digested foods that can be obtained for this purpose.

The carbohydrates which occur in our foods chiefly as sugars and starches are combinations of the chemical elements of carbon, hydrogen, and oxygen. These foods are broken down during the digestive process into simple sugars absorbed into the blood. It is from the blood that the tissue cells can withdraw sugar according to their energy needs.

Our main source of carbohydrates is foods composed of grains. These include breads and cereals (some of which are also rich in protein, minerals, and vitamins), spaghetti, macaroni, pastries, and the like. Potatoes are also a major source of starch, but they contain other important food values as well.

Of course the carbohydrate foods are an important source of the total diet, but a great many people consume them in excess and at the expense of other perhaps less abundant and more needed foods. From infancy numerous people are actually trained to be especially fond of candies and dessert foods since these are used by parents as a reward for "cleaning up" one's plate, eating unwanted foods, and being "good" in other ways. In excess of bodily needs, such high energy foods have been termed "empty calories," because they provide little or nothing of value. Indeed, they well encourage fatness while at the same time satisfying the appetite when other food values are needed. It is not suggested that an effort be made to eliminate pastries and candies from the diet, but an effort should be made to reduce their prominence, especially among the less active. After all, fruits, vegetables, and juices can be equally satisfying snack and dessert foods which are relatively low in calories and high in other nutrients, and they do not confront the body with the problem of disposing of pure, unneeded energy.

Generally speaking, usable carbohydrates have at least two fates in the body. The first, and most relevant to stress, is the formation of glucose. Glucose is the major energy source for the body and the only form of energy used by the brain, nerves and lung tissue. One gram of carbohydrate yields four calories of energy. The second fate of carbohydrates is the formation of glycogen from glucose. Glycogen is a form of stored energy with the principal stores being in the liver. Smaller reserves are found in the muscles. Blood glucose comes from dietary complex carbohydrates and simple carbohydrates. During a typical stress response extra blood glucose to take care of the emergency (real or imagined) is supplied by the breakdown of glycogen into glucose.[14]

Fats

Fats are derived from the same chemical elements as carbohydrates, but the combination of the carbon, hydrogen, and oxygen is different. Fats contain more carbon but less oxygen than carbohydrates, and they are a more concentrated energy source than either carbohydrates or proteins. They also contribute to the bodily functioning in other important ways and should not, therefore, be considered as substances to be eliminated entirely from the diet.

Fat deposits in the body serve as insulation and shock absorption material and as reserve energy in storage. Individuals whose energy expenditure is likely to exceed that provided by their carbohydrate intake are especially in need of some of the "slower burning" fats in their diet. Individuals who wish or need to reduce their weight or who have certain circulatory disorders and risks are usually advised to restrict their fat intake more or less sharply.

Minerals

The mineral elements of the body are often referred to as ash constituents, for they are the residue left from the oxidation process of the organic compounds which we eat in the form of food. In simpler terms, we may liken them to the ashes which remain after the burning of wood or coal. The mineral elements compose about four percent of the total body weight with calcium accounting for approximately two of the four percent.

Included among the minerals are calcium, phosphorus, potassium, sulfur, chlorine, sodium, magnesium, iron, iodine, manganese, copper, cobalt, nickel, and flourine. The majority of the minerals are needed in minute quantities that are plentiful in a good diet. However, calcium, iron, and iodine are needed in appreciable quantities and therefore may require special consideration in the diet.

The major functions of minerals in the body are to serve as building and regulatory substances. As structural constituents they operate in three general ways: (1) they give rigidity to the hard tissues of the bones and teeth, (2) they serve as components of soft tissues in muscle and nerve, and (3) they often serve as the crucial element necessary for the production of hormones such as iodine in thyroxin. As a regulator of body processes, minerals serve in many ways, examples of which are: (1) they (calcium) are essential for the coagulation of the blood, (2) they protect against the accumulation of too much acid or alkali in the blood and body tissues, (3) they are involved in the maintenance of the normal rhythm of the heartbeat, (4) they aid in the exchange of water in the tissues, and (5) they are involved in the transmission of nerve impulses.

Minerals have an important and diverse use in human metabolism. Since many of them are required in carbohydrate, fat, and protein metabolism, they would be important in the energy reaction required during the stress response. However, it is important to take minerals in balanced proportions and not in excessive amounts since they can be toxic in high doses.[14]

Vitamins

From an historical point of view, the realization that vitamins are basic nutrients stands as a milestone in the emergence of the field of nutrition as a scientifically-based discipline. Unlike such nutrients as proteins, fats, and minerals, vitamins do not become a part of the structure of the body, but rather they serve as catalysts which make possible various chemical reactions within the body. These reactions have to do with converting food substances into the elements needed for utilization by the various cells of the body. For example, vitamin D needs to be present if calcium is to be metabolized and made available for use in the blood and bones.

The vitamins with which we are familiar today are commonly classified as fat soluble or water soluble. This designation means that the one group requires fatty substances and the other water if they are to be dissolved and used by the body. Although a large number of vitamins have been identified as being important to human nutrition, the exact function of many of them has not as yet been determined.

In countries such as the United States it should not be difficult for people to select a diet which is sufficiently varied to include all necessary vitamins. However, poor dietary practices can lead to vitamin inadequacy, and as a precaution many people supplement their diets with vitamin pills. Even though such a supplement may not be needed, when taken in small amounts the vitamins may do no harm. This is particularly true of the water soluble vitamins in that if one gets more than needed they will pass right through the body. (Recently, some scientists have been disputing this claim, especially if water soluble vitamins are taken in extra large doses.) On the other hand, some of the fat soluble vitamins may be toxic and overdoses could render possible harm. Of course, extra vitamins may be prescribed by physicians for a variety of reasons.

In recent years a great deal of controversy has emerged as a result of what has been called *megavitamin therapy*, which concerns the use of certain vitamins in massive doses — sometimes as much as one thousand times the U.S. Recommended Daily Allowance. The proponents for megavitamin therapy believe that massive doses of such vitamins, particularly vitamin C, and in some cases the B complex vitamins, will prevent certain diseases and very significantly extend life. On the contrary, opponents of the practice maintain that it not only may be useless, but in some instances harmful as well.

It is interesting to note that there is support in some quarters for massive dosages of certain vitamins as an important factor in surviving stress. In fact, there is a classification of vitamins sold over the counter which are called *stress formula vitamins*, and they go by a variety of brand names. The formula for these is one which includes large amounts of vitamin C and vitamin B complex. Anyone contemplating utilizing a vitamin supplement over and above the U.S. Recommended Daily Allowance should do so in consultation with a physician and/or a qualified nutritionist.

Water

Human beings are about 71 percent water by weight, and this water, evaporating and flowing from the surface of the body, and breathed out as vapor on the breath, must be continuously replenished if one is to remain alive. The chemical changes which make life possible can take place only in solution, and it is water which provides the necessary solvent.

The body secures the water which it needs from fluids taken as drink, from foods which are eaten, and from the water formed by the combustion of foods in the body. The body loses water in the form of urine from the kidneys, fecal discharge from the intestinal tract, perspiration from the skin, and exhaled breath from the lungs.

Physical activity, environmental heat, and the normal bodily processes lead more or less rapidly to water loss. If this loss is not balanced by water intake, dehydration can occur. For short periods this loss is harmless and leads to thirst and restoration of normal water level and body weight with copious drinking. However, if the dehydrated state continues over an extended period of time, bodily functions become seriously jeopardized since water is involved in all of them.

Arbitrary recommendations have been made concerning the desirable water intake per day. However, there are so many factors which affect the need for it — factors such as the fluid content of other liquids in food, how active a person is, and the environmental temperature — that we are inclined to recommend your thirst as a guide.

Calories

Many people labor under the misconception that a calorie is a nutrient just like fats, carbohydrates, or proteins. Actually, a calorie is a unit of measurement just like an ounce or an inch. The body requires energy to function and heat is the by-product of this energy. A calorie is the amount of heat necessary to raise the temperature of one kilogram (2.2 pounds) of water one degree centigrade. Since food is our source of fuel, scientists have been interested in computing the number of calories which different foods provide, as well as the number of calories which the body must utilize in the performance of various activities. The results of these studies have furnished information which tells us how many calories or heat units the food we eat must produce in order to provide us with enough energy to meet our needs. These energy needs may be classified into two categories, those that are voluntary and those that are involuntary. Voluntary activities are those over which we have control, but the involuntary energy demands are those which take place continously whether we are awake or asleep. Among the latter are digestion, heart function, elimination, breathing, and such special demands automatically brought on by emotional excitation, stress, and environmental heat.

The energy needed to sustain all bodily functions when one is at "complete rest" is known as the *basal metabolism*. The basal metabolic rate (B.M.R.) is computed by measuring the amount of oxygen which is consumed by a person after lying at rest for a given period of time. The oxygen which is consumed is indicative of the number of calories of heat which is produced. The BMR is then translated by means of a formula into the number of calories per square meter of the body surface per hours of rest.

An individual's BMR when at rest and when doing various amounts of physical activity can give a good indication of the amount of effort that is going into the work that one is doing — work, that is, just to maintain life at rest or heavy physical work, as the case may be.

Digestion

The digestive system of the body is more than 30 feet long from beginning to end, and the chemical processes that occur within the walls of this mucus-lined hollow tube are extremely complex in nature. From the moment that food is taken into the mouth until waste products are excreted, the body's chemical laboratory is at work. The principal parts of this system are the alimentary canal, consisting of the oral cavity, pharnyx, esophagus, stomach, small intestine, and large intestine. Two additional organs are necessary to complete the digestive system. These are the liver and the pancreas, both of which connect to the small intestine. It is from these two organs that many of the essentially digestive juices are secreted.

As mentioned previously, the function of the digestive system is to change the composition of foods which we ingest. Reduced to simpler chemical substances, the foods can be readily absorbed through the lining of the intestines for distribution by the circulatory system to the millions of body cells. These end products of digestion are in the form of simple sugars, fatty acids, amino acids, minerals, and vitamins.

Digestion is also accomplished by mechanical action. First, the food is broken down by the grinding action of the teeth. This increases tremendously the food surface area upon which the various digestive juices can act. It is then swallowed and eventually is moved through the alimentary canal by a process called peristalsis. This is a series of muscular contractions, which mix the contents of the digestive tract and keep it on the move.

The digestive tract is exceedingly responsive to one's emotional state. Food eaten under happy conditions tend to be readily digested. On the contrary, digestion may be impeded and even stopped for a considerable period of time (as much as a day or more) if severe emotional stress occurs. Extensive nerve connections in the digestive tract tend to make its organs especially susceptible to disorders caused by stress. Examples of some of these disorders are nausea, diarrhea, and colitis (inflammation of the large bowel). In such disorders the organs involved may not necessarily be diseased and there may only be an impaired functioning of the organ. However, many authorities agree that prolonged emotional stress can lead to serious diseases of the digestive tract. Two of my associates on a stress project, Drs. Donald Morse and Robert Pollack,[14] contend that stress is the principal reason for digestive disturbances. For example, in their work on stress and saliva, it has been found that stress causes dry mouth. This is particularly important since digestion starts in the mouth and saliva is needed to start the digestion of starch.

There is a popular belief that a bowel movement per day is essential to health. Moreover, so common rumor has it, to be really effective, this movement should occur at a particular time each day. "Autointoxication" or self-poisoning, it is sometimes claimed, may otherwise result. As a matter of fact, many people do find a bowel movement once a day satisfactory and having it at a particular time, convenient. However, just as some require more than one elimination per day, others find every other day a natural rhythm—and not a cause of constipation (a condition that has Americans spending nearly a billion dollars annually on laxatives). Thus, the problem is not one of conforming to an arbitrary standard, but discovering one's own natural rhythm and responding to the urge when it comes.

DIET

The term *diet* is an all inclusive one to refer to foods and liquids regularly consumed. The question often raised is: "What constitutes a balanced diet?" This means essentially, that along with sufficient fluids, one should include foods from the *four basic food groups*. These are the dairy group, the meat group, the vegetable and fruit group, and the bread and cereal group.

A guide to a balanced diet was prepared by the staff of the United States Senate Select Committee on Nutrition and Human Needs. This Committee spent a great deal of time on hearings and research and some of its recommendations are listed as follows:

1. Eat less meat and more fish and poultry.
2. Replace whole milk with skim milk.
3. Reduce intake of eggs, butter, and other high-cholestrol sources.
4. Cut back on sugars to 15 percent of daily caloric intake.
5. Reduce intake of salt to a total of three grams per day.
6. Eat more fruit, vegetables, and whole grain.

The above recommendations are directed to the general population. However, one important fact must be remembered, and this is that eating is an individual matter. The problem may not be so much one of following an arbitrary diet, but one of learning to know on what foods and proportions of foods one functions best. The body is capable of compensating for an imbalance in the nutrients which one fails to get if the shortage is made up within a reasonable period of time. In other words, it is not necessary to have an exactly balanced diet at every meal. Indeed, it is possible to miss meals — even go for several days without food — and show no signs of malnutrition. The important consideration seems to be in the quality of the total intake over periods of time.

The foregoing observations should *not* be interpreted to mean that one should be indifferent or careless about food choices. After all, you quite literally *are* what you eat. And, it is absurd that some people are more careful about what they feed their pets than they are about what they eat themselves. This kind of thoughtlessness has given rise to the claim that Americans are the most overfed *and* malnourished people in the world. Any radical departure from one's diet should be made only under the guidance of a physician and/or a qualified nutritionist.

It was mentioned previously that you are quite literally what you eat. This old adage has recently been brought more clearly into focus because researchers now know that our bodies synthesize food substances known as *neurotransmitters*. Prominent nutritionists tend to be of the opinion that these neurotransmitters relay messages to the brain which, in turn, affect our moods, sex drive, appetite, and even personality. This is to say that adding a certain food or omitting another could be just what a person might need. It is believed that when a person is stressed, the body becomes less able to use protein. Therefore, the general recommendation is that after any kind of stress one should eat more lean meat, fish, or milk products. Also, since stress depletes the supply of vitamin C and potassium, these should be replaced by eating extra portions of citrus products.

The diets of some families include too much of certain foods that can be potentially harmful. A case in point is the intake of *cholesterol*. Excessive amounts of this chemical component of animal oils and fats are deposited in blood vessels and may be a factor in the causation of hardening of the arteries leading to a heart attack.

In his interesting book *The Healing Heart*, Norman Cousins[5] suggests that the accumulation of these fatty substances is not something that begins in upper middle age. On the contrary, the process can begin in early childhood. A 1982 – 1983 study of children in New York City and Los Angeles conducted by Dr. Ernest L. Wynder of the American Heart Foundation showed average cholesterol levels of 180 for children in the

10 to 12 age range. Continuing on the same course would lead to cholesterol levels close to, or about 300 by the age of 35. (Physicians vary widely in their beliefs about safe levels of cholesterol; however, some use a very broad range of 150 to 300 as being normal, the average of this range being 225.)

Diet and Weight Control

Basically, weight gain or loss is a matter of energy intake versus energy expenditure of the body. If one wishes to decrease body fat he or she can reduce caloric intake (which is most easily done by reducing the amount of high energy foods) and energy expenditure can be increased by means of pleasurable physical activity. By doing both one can lower weight in a given amount of time by less severe dieting than would otherwise be necessary to accomplish the same thing.

Since dieting is the most popular way of controlling weight in this country it seems appropriate that certain general principles should be established when one undertakes the practice. The following list of such principles was developed by one of my former associates, the late Dr. Warren Johnson[10] and might well be considered by one who is contemplating a weight control program.

1. The advisability of getting a physician's advice is emphasized.
2. If fat is to be lost, the calories taken in must be fewer than those needed for the body's energy requirements.
3. The diet, though low in calories, is adequate in all other nutrients so that intakes for these do not become dangerously low.
4. It should be recognized that losing weight is not easy.
5. Foods are not forbidden but portion control is emphasized.
6. There is a sensible balance of energy-providing nutrients.
7. The diet is realistic and does not call for superhuman effort.
8. Exercise at the same time is recommended.
9. The behaviors and emotions that lead to eating are examined, and advice is given to help the dieter control these.

Diet and Stress

With very few exceptions, writers on the subject of stress emphasize the importance of diet as a general health measure. However, the question to pose is: "Are there any specific forms of diet that can contribute to the prevention of stress and/or help one cope with it?"

One specific approach to diet and stress is presented by Dr. J. Daniel Palm[15] who suggests that many stress-related disorders are related to problems which originate in the regulation of the blood sugar level.

Dr. Palm's theory, developed as an extension of the data derived from controlled research, states that an insufficiency of sugar in the blood supplied to the brain is enough of a detrimental condition, and therefore a stress, to initiate physiological responses and behavioral changes which develop into a variety of disorders. A deficiency of blood sugar which is known to be associated with various disorders is seen not as a consequence of the disease but as a primary and original physiological stress. Behavior changes may be inadequate or inappropriate attempts of the stress-affected persons to compensate. It is believed that if the stress of an insufficiency of blood sugar can be prevented various kinds of abnormal behavior can be controlled. To eliminate this stress of a deficiency of blood sugar a new dietary program is proposed by Dr. Palm. This diet is based on the metabolic characteristics of *fructose* (fruit sugar) and its advantageous use when it is exchanged for glucose or other carbohydrates which are digested to glucose and then absorbed. (Fructose itself is a normal constituent of sucrose, which is ordinary table sugar. It also occurs naturally in many fruits and constitutes half the content of honey.)

Practically all theories have enthusiastic proponents as well as equally unenthusiastic opponents, and this sometimes results in a great deal of confusion among most of us. The fact that the human organism is so complicated and complex make any kind of research connected with it extremely difficult. Nevertheless, scholars in the scientific community continue to make important inquiries into the study of human needs. It is emphasized again, and forcefully, that individuals concerned in any way with their own specific dietary problems should consult a physician and/or a qualified nutritionist for guidance.

REST AND SLEEP

To be effective on the job and to enjoy leisure to the utmost, periodic recuperation is an essential ingredient in daily living patterns. Rest and sleep provide us with the means of revitalizing ourselves to meet the challenges of our responsibilities.

The nature of stress is such that it imposes a tremendous drain on the organism and hastens fatigue. (Chronic and acute aspects of fatigue were discussed in Chapter Four.) In order to keep fatigue at a minimum and in its proper proportion in the cycle of everyday activities, nature has provided us with ways to combat and reduce it in the form of rest and sleep.

Rest and sleep are essential to life as they afford the body the chance to regain its vitality and efficiency in a very positive way. Learning to utilize opportunities for rest and sleep may add years to our lives and zest to our years. Although rest and sleep are closely allied, they are not synonymous. For this reason it is appropriate to consider them separately.

Rest

In general, most people think of rest as just "taking it easy." A chief purpose of rest is to reduce tension so that the body may be better able to recover from fatigue. There is no overt activity involved, but neither is there loss of consciousness as in sleep. In rest, there is not loss of awareness of the external environment as in sleep. Since the need for rest is usually in direct proportion to the type of activity in which we engage, it follows naturally that the more strenuous the activity, the more frequent the rest periods should be. A busy day on the job may not be noticeably active as a game of tennis, nevertheless, it is the wise person who will let the body dictate when a rest period is required. Five or ten minutes of sitting in a chair with the eyes closed may make the difference in the course of an active day, assuming of course that this is possible. The real effectiveness of rest periods depends largely on the individual and his or her ability to let down and rest. (Nurses under severe stress may find this very difficult to accomplish.)

Sleep

Sleep is a phenomenon that has never been clearly defined or understood but has aptly been named the "great restorer." It is no wonder that authorities on the subject agree that sleep is essential to the vital functioning of the body and that natural sleep is the most satisfying form of recuperation from fatigue. It is during the hours of sleep that the body is given an opportunity to revitalize itself. All vital functions are slowed down so that the building of new cells and the repair of tissues can take place without undue interruption. This does not mean that the body builds and regenerates tissue only during sleep, but it does mean that it is the time that nature has set aside to accomplish the task more easily. The body's metabolic rate is lowered and energy is restored.

Despite the acknowledged need for sleep, a question of paramount importance concerns the amount of sleep necessary for the body to accomplish its recuperative task. There is no clear-cut answer to this query. Sleep is an individual matter, based on degree rather than kind. The usual recommendation for adults is eight hours of sleep out of every 24, but the basis for this could well be one of fallacy rather than fact. There are many persons who can function effectively on less sleep, while others require more. No matter how many hours of sleep you get during the course of a 24-hour period, perhaps the best test of adequacy will depend largely on how you feel. If you are normally alert, feel healthy, and are in good humor, you are probably getting a sufficient amount of sleep. The rest that sleep normally brings to the body depends to a large extent upon a person's freedom from excessive emotional stress and ability to relax. Unrelaxed sleep has little restorative value, but learning to relax is a skill that is not acquired in one night.

Is loss of sleep dangerous? This is a question that is pondered quite frequently. Again, the answer is not simple. To the normally healthy person with normal sleep habits, an occasional missing of the accustomed hours is not serious. On the other hand, repeated loss of sleep over a period of time can be dangerous. It is the loss of sleep night after night, rather than at one time, that apparently does the damage and results in the condition previously described as chronic fatigue. The general effects of loss of sleep are likely to result in poor general health, nervousness, irritability, inability to concentrate, lowered perseverance of effort, and serious fatigue. Studies have shown that a person can go for much longer periods of time without food than without sleep. In some instances successive loss of sleep for long periods has proven fatal. Under normal conditions, however, a night of lost sleep followed by a period of prolonged sleep will restore the individual to his or her normal self.

There are many conditions that tend to rob the body of restful slumber. Most certainly, mental anguish and worry play a very large part in holding sleep at bay. Some factors that influence the quality of sleep are hunger, cold, boredom, and excessive fatigue. In many instances these factors can be controlled. Incidentally, Dr. Robert Coursey,[4] a psychologist at the University of Maryland and a researcher of sleep, has indicated that people who are "insomniacs" may only think they are, and one of the things that insomniacs worry about incessively is their sleepless condition. His definition of a chronic insomniac is one who takes longer to fall asleep, has more trouble staying asleep, wakes up earlier than a normal sleeper and feels tired as a result. In any case, insomnia and chronic fatigue might well be brought to the attention of a physician so that the necessary steps can be taken to bring about restoration of normal sleep patterns. Certainly, drugs to induce sleep should be utilized only if prescribed by a physician. (A few of the nurse respondents in my survey said they used tranquilizers to combat stress and these were about equally divided between prescribed and over-the-counter drugs.)

Many recommendations about sleep have been made by authoritative sources and some of these are cited here. One source [3] suggests techniques that will help are relaxing physically and mentally before retiring, reducing your tension level during the day, and managing your time, activities, and thoughts to prepare for a good night's sleep. Another source [13] recommends that the process should be the same each night, and should begin at the same hour, leading to repose at the same time. That is, if your bedtime is normally eleven o'clock your preparation should begin by at least ten and not later than ten-thirty. If work has been brought home, you should break off at least one-half hour before the fixed retirement time; and, during this half-hour, stimulants should be avoided, but a glass of warm milk can be an excellent tranquilizer.

Understanding the complex nature of sleep may be the province of scientists and other qualified experts, but an understanding of the value of sleep is the responsibility of everyone.

PHYSICAL ACTIVITY AND EXERCISE

The proportion of my nurse respondents indicating that they engage in some sort of physical activity and exercise to combat stress was somewhat less than other populations I have studied. Although several nurses engaged in certain physical activities, at the same time most said it was done on a more or less sporadic and spasmodic basis. Many professed that they should be on some sort of regular exercise program.

When used in connection with the human organism, the term *physical* means a concern for the body and its needs. The term *activity* derives from the word *active*, one meaning of which is the requirement of action. Thus, when the two words physical and activity are used together, it implies body action. This is a broad term and could include any voluntary and/or involuntary body movement. When such body movement is practiced for the purpose of developing and maintaining physical fitness, it is ordinarily referred to as physical *exercise*. This section of the chapter is concerned with both the broad area of physical activity and the more specific area of physical exercise, and will take into account how these factors are concerned with all around health as well as how they relate to stress.

The Physical Aspect of Personality

One point of departure in discussing the physical aspect of personality could be to state that "everybody has a body." Some are short, some are tall, some are lean, and some are fat. People (including nurses) come in different sizes, but all of them have a certain innate capacity that is influenced by the environment.

As far as human beings are concerned—from early childhood through adulthood—it might be said that the body is our base of operation, what could be called our "physical base." The other components of the total personality—social, emotional, and intellectual—are somewhat vague. Although these are manifested in various ways, we do not actually see them as we do the physical aspect. Consequently, it becomes all important that starting as children, that a serious attempt be made to gain control over the physical aspect or what is known as basic body control. The ability to do this, of course, will vary from one person to another. It will depend to a large extent upon our status of physical fitness.

The broad area of physical fitness can be broken down into certain components, and it is important that individuals achieve to the best of their natural ability as far as these components are concerned. There is not complete agreement as far as identification of the components of physical fitness are concerned. However, the following information provided by the President's Council on Physical Fitness and Sports[16] considers certain components to be basic:

1. *Muscular strength*. This refers to the contraction power of muscles. The strength of muscles is usually measured with dynamometers or tensiometers, which record the amount of force particular muscle groups can apply in a single maximum effort. All movements of the body or any of its parts are impossible without action by muscles attached to the skeleton. Muscles perform vital functions of the body as well. The heart is a muscle; death occurs when it ceases to contract. Breathing, digestion, and elimination are dependent upon muscular contractions. These vital muscular functions are in-

fluenced by exercising the skeletal muscles; the heart beats faster, the blood circulates through the body at a greater rate, breathing becomes deep and rapid, and perspiration breaks out on the surface of the skin.

2. *Muscular endurance*. Muscular endurance is the ability of muscles to perform work. Two variations of muscular endurance are recognized: *isotonic*, whereby the muscles continue to raise and lower a submaximal load as in weight training or performing push-ups. In the *isometric* form, the muscles maintain a fixed length; in the isotonic form, they alternately shorten and lengthen. Muscular endurance must assume some muscular strength. However, there are distinctions between the two; muscle groups of the same strength may possess different degrees of endurance.

3. *Circulatory-respiratory endurance*. Circulatory-respiratory endurance is characterized by moderate contractions of large muscle groups for relatively long periods of time, during which maximal adjustments of the circulatory-respiratory system to the activity are necessary, as in distance running and swimming. Obviously, strong and enduring muscles are needed. However, by themselves they are not enough; they do not guarantee well-developed circulatory-respiratory functions.

As far as the physical aspect of personality is concerned, a major objective of modern man and woman should be directed to maintaining a suitable level of physical fitness, the topic of the ensuing discussion.

Maintaining a Suitable Level of Physical Fitness

Physical fitness presupposes an adequate intake of good food and an adequate amount of rest and sleep, but beyond these things, activity involving all the big muscles of the body is essential. Just how high a level of physical fitness should be maintained from one stage of life to another is a difficult question to answer because we must raise the question: "Fitness for what?" Obviously, the young varsity athlete needs to think of a level of fitness far above that which will concern the average middle-aged individual.

Physical fitness has been described in different ways by different people; however, when all of these descriptions are put together it is likely that they will be characterized more by their similarities than by their differences. For my purpose I will think of physical fitness as the level of ability of the human organism to perform certain physical tasks, or put another way, the fitness to perform various specified tasks requiring muscular effort.

The word *exercise* may tend to have strong moralistic overtones. Like so many things that are said to be "good for you," it also tends to give rise to certain feelings of boredom and resentment. Thus, many people draw more than facetious pleasure in repeating such old sayings as: "When I feel like exercising, I lie down quickly until the feeling goes away," and "I get my exercise serving as pall-bearer for my friends who exercised."

Exercising and maintaining some level of physical fitness makes possible types of meaningful experiences in life that are not otherwise available to you. These experiences include all manner of physical activities and exercise, including indoor and outdoor sports; and they also include the rich and satisfying interpersonal relationships that are usually associated with these activities.

Types of Exercises

For discussion here I will consider three types of exercises: (1) *proprioceptive-facilitative,* (2) *isotonic,* and (3) *isometric.*

Proprioceptive-Facilitative Exercises

These exercises are those that consist of various refined patterns of movement found in most team games and individual sports. Various combinations of the following features are involved in the performance of this type of exercise:

1. *Muscular power.* Ability to release maximum force in the shortest time.
2. *Agility.* Speed in changing body position or in changing direction.
3. *Speed.* Rapidity with which successive movements of the same kind can be performed.
4. *Flexibility.* Range of movement in a joint or a sequence of joints.
5. *Balance.* Ability to maintain position and equilibrium both in movement (dynamic balance) and while stationary (static balance).
6. *Coordination.* Working together of the muscles and organs of the human body in the performance of a specific task.

Isotonic Exercises

An isotonic exercise involves the amount of resistance one can overcome during one application of force through the full range of motion in a given joint or joints. An example of this would be picking up a weight and flexing the elbows while lifting the weight to shoulder height.

Isotonic exercises can improve strength to some extent. They are also very useful for increasing and maintaining full range of motion. Such range of motion should be maintained throughout life if possible although it can decrease with age and with such musculoskeletal disorders as arthritis. This disease can cause shortening of fibrous tissue structure and this is likely to limit the normal range of motion.

Another important feature of isotonic exercise is that it can increase circulatory-respiratory endurance in such activities as running and swimming. (Incidentally, swimming was a favorite of many of the nurses in my survey.)

Isometric Exercises

Although isometrics do not provide much in the way of improvement of normal range of motion and endurance, they are most useful in increasing strength and volume of muscles. In isometrics, the muscle is contracted, but the length of the muscle is generally the same during contraction as during relaxation. The contraction is accomplished by keeping two joints rigid while at the same time contracting the muscle(s) between the joints. A maximal amount of force is applied against a fixed resistance during one all-out effort. An example of this is pushing and pulling against an immovable object. Let us say that if you place your hands against a wall and push with as much force as you can, you have effected the contraction of certain muscles while their length has remained essentially the same. (Several of these types of exercises will be recommended later in the chapter.)

Developing Your Own Program

One of the problems of most nurses is that they are not likely to have available services and facilities designed for participation in regularly planned physical activities. However, a few nurses in my survey indicated that they held memberships in various forms of health clubs. It seems appropriate to consider some of those factors that are concerned with embarking on a program.

The traditional recommendation has been to consult a physician before undertaking a physical activity program. However, a recent publication[6] by the National Heart, Lung, and Blood Institute — the government agency that finances much of the heart disease research —

tends to dispel this notion. The position is taken that failing to exercise regularly can be far more dangerous than by abstaining because one may not be willing to consult a doctor first. In fact, several in the field of public health tend to believe that not seeing a doctor first may be preventing millions of people from starting an exercise program. My own position is that it is a personal matter as to whether or not one should consult a physician before embarking on a physical activity program. If a person feels more comfortable by consulting a doctor first, then perhaps he or she should do so. It is likely that a physician will recommend the program without restriction, or if a physical problem is found, the doctor will take steps to correct it — and there may be suggestions for modifying the program to make it more suitable to the particular individual.

The next consideration is that a program be an individual matter and one that fits your own needs and wishes. In other words, if a person is not happy with the program, it will be unlikely that it will meet with success as far as personal goals are concerned. Each individual will have to determine which particular approach is best for him or her, specified physical exercises, recreational sports, or a combination of both.

Once you have decided what you are going to do for your exercise program, whether prescribed exercises or recreational sports, you will need to determine how many times a week to engage in these activities. It is best to avoid the extremes of the "once in a while" or "always without fail" spurts and try to maintain a regular schedule of three to four times a week. It is also a good idea to work out on alternate days — Monday, Wednesday, and Friday, or Tuesday, Thursday, and Saturday. The hour of the day does not necessarily matter. However, it should be remembered that if you have already decided that your fitness program is going to be number one on your list of priorities, it should not be difficult to get into the habit of putting regular workouts into your weekly schedule.

IMPORTANCE OF PHYSICAL EXERCISE
IN REDUCING STRESS

The value of exercise as a means of reducing stress is well documented by various sources. According to Walter McQuade and Ann Aikman,[12] one of the many stresses people suffer from is stress resulting from their own pent-up aggressive drives. When people express these drives in physical action, they are better off because exercise not only dispels this form of stress, but also it enables the body to hold up better against stress in general.

Similarly, Beata Jencks[9] reports that physical and emotional trauma upset balance of body and mind, and that much energy is wasted in muscular tension, bringing on unnecessary tiredness and exhaustion. If stress reactions become habit patterns, then the muscles and tendons shorten and thicken and excessive connective tissue is deposited, causing a general consolidation of tissues. She comments further that excess energy, released by action of the sympathetic nervous system, if not immediately dissipated by muscular action, produces muscular or nervous tension and that this tension should be dissipated by muscular action in the form of exercise.

From a genetic point of view, C. Eugene Walker[18] suggests that exercise is very effective in reducing anxiety, although he states that how this occurs is not entirely understood. It may be that it satisfies the evolutionary need of man to engage in large muscle, physically aggressive activity that was very adaptive for primitive man, but with our highly civilized, sedentary, and confined lifestyle, has fewer acceptable outlets. He concludes that whatever the basis for it, exercise does have an anxiety- and tension-reducing effect. People on exercise programs tend to be more healthy, have better vital capacity, handle problems better, sleep better, and cope with life in general in a more satisfactory way. Thus, exercise immediately reduces anxiety somewhat and over the long run tends to inoculate against the development of future anxieties.

As far as objective evidence and scientific inquiry is concerned, a number of controlled studies are currently providing findings that show that physical activity contributes to our capacity to reduce stress.

Activities for Stressful Situations

Many occupations and professions (and certainly nursing) produce various kinds of stressful conditions, and many of these occur in the immediate environment. The foregoing discussion has focused on the importance of physical activity in helping one deal with stress. The present discussion is concerned with the worker's active behavior in a stressful situation. More specifically, what can you as a nurse do in the way of physical activity to deal with a stressful situation in the immediate environment?

Various authentic pronouncements have been made that support the idea that instant activity can be beneficial. For example, Reuven Gal and Richard Lazarus[7] report that being engaged in activity — rather than remaining passive — is preferable in most individuals in most stressful situations and can be highly effective in reducing threat and distress. The latter[11] has also maintained that a person may alter his or her psychological and physiological stress reactions in a given situation simply by taking action, and this in turn, will affect his or her appraisal of the situation, thereby ultimately altering the stress reaction.

What then are some of the physical activities that one can engage in as a reaction to a stressful situation? Obviously, it would not be appropriate to engage in isotonics by dropping to the floor and doing pushups or to break into a two-mile jog around the room. Isometrics are recommended for this purpose and they can be peformed in a more or less subtle manner and not necessarily be noticed by others. I have developed the following possibilities and certainly creative nurses will be able to think of others.

1. *Hand and Head Press.* Interweave fingers and place hands at the back of the head with elbows pointing out. Push the head backward on the hands while simultaneously pulling the head forward with the hands. Although this can be done while standing, it can also be done while sitting at a desk or table and is less conspicuous.
2. *Wall Press.* Stand with the back against the wall. Allow the arms to hang down at the sides. Turn hands toward the wall and press the wall with the palms, keeping the arms straight.
3. *Hand Pull.* Bend the right elbow and bring the right hand in with the palm up close to the front of the body. Put the left hand in the right hand. Try to curl the right arm upward while simultaneously resisting with the left hand. Repeat using the opposite pressure. This can be done while standing or sitting at a desk or table.
4. *Hand Push.* The hands are clasped with the palms together close to the chest with the elbows pointing out. Press the hands together firmly.
5. *Leg Press.* While sitting at a desk or table, cross the left ankle over the right ankle. The feet are on the floor and the legs are at about a right angle. Try to straighten the right leg while resisting with the left leg. Repeat with the right ankle over the left ankle.
6. *The Gripper.* Place one hand in the other and grip hard. Another variation is to grip an object. While standing, this could be the back of a chair or, while sitting, it could be the arms of a chair or the seat.
7. *Chair Push.* While sitting at a desk or table with the hands on the

armrests of the chair, push down with the hands. The entire buttocks can be raised from the chair seat. One or both feet can be lifted
off the floor, or both can remain in contact with the floor.

8. *Hip Lifter.* While sitting at a desk or table, lift one buttock after the
   other from the chair seat. Try to keep the head from moving. The
   hands can be placed at the sides of the chair seat for balance.

9. *Heel and Toe.* From a standing position, rise on the toes. Come back
   down on the heels while raising both the toes and the balls of the feet.

10. *Fist Clencher.* Clench fists and then open hands extending the fingers
    as far as possible.

This short list is comprised of representative examples of isometric
exercises, and they are actually referred to by some as *stress exercises.*
While it has been recommended that these types of activities can be performed easily in the work environment, it is obvious that they can be
performed elsewhere as well. Wherever they are performed it might be
well to observe the following recommendations of the President's Council on Physical Fitness.[1]

One hard six-to-eight second isometric contraction per workout can
over a period of six months, produce a significant strength increase in a
muscle. There is no set order for doing isometric exercises — nor does a
whole series have to be completed at one time. For each contraction,
maintain tension for not more than eight seconds. Do little breathing
during the contraction; breath deeply between contractions. Start easily,
and do not apply maximum effort in the beginning. For the first three or
four weeks one should exert only about one-half of what is the maximum
force. Use the first three or four seconds to build up this degree of
force — and the remaining four or five seconds to hold it.

I have recommended these isometric exercises to many nurses I have
known. They have had good success with them in their particular work
environment; and I hope you will too!

It seems appropriate to conclude this chapter with a statement from
the "Father of Stress," my friend, the late Hans Selye.[17]

> Physical activity is an excellent way to relieve the pressures bearing
> on our minds and to equalize the wear and tear throughout the body,
> giving overworked parts a time to rest. Most people seek diversion in-
> tuitively for these reasons, just as an athlete may read for relaxation,
> the sedentary man may engage in sports for a change of pace. The rich
> executive, although he would not dream of relaxing by moving heavy
> furniture, may enjoy a regular workout in his club's gym. Further-
> more, we must not forget that while exercising is beneficial in reducing

stress, it also helps us combat the physical decay of aging—indeed, this is one of the reasons I used to race about the university on my bicycle each morning.

REFERENCES

1. *Adult Physical Fitness*, Washington, D.C., U.S. Government Printing Office, 1976.
2. Berland, Theodore. The Diet Connection, *Insider*, November, 1977.
3. Coates, Thomas J., and Carl E. Thoresen. *How to Sleep Better*, Englewood Cliffs, NJ, Prentice-Hall, Inc., 1977.
4. Coursey, Robert D. To Sleep or Not to Sleep—That is the Problem, *Precis*, College Park, MD, September 12, 1977.
5. Cousins, Norman, *The Healing Heart*, New York, W.W. Norton and Company, 1983.
6. *Exercise and Your Heart*, Consumer Information Center, Dept. P, Pueblo, CO.
7. Gal, Reuven and Richard S. Lazarus. The Role of Activity in Anticipating and Confronting Stressful Situations, *Journal of Human Stress*, December, 1975.
8. Gonzales, Nick. What's Eating You? *Family Health*, November, 1977.
9. Jencks, Beata. *Your Body Biofeedback at Its Best*, Chicago, Nelson-Hall, Inc., 1977.
10. Johnson, Warren R. *Health in Action*, New York, Holt, Rinehart and Winston, 1977.
11. Lazarus, Richard S. The Self-Regulation of Emotion, New York, Raven Press, 1975, L. Levy (ed.), *Parameters of Emotion.*
12. McQuade, Walter and Ann Aikman. *Stress*, New York, E.P. Dutton and Co., Inc., 1974.
13. Morehouse, Laurence E. and Leonard Gross. *Total Fitness in Thirty Minutes a Week*, New York, Simon and Schuster, 1975.
14. Morse, Donald R. and Robert L. Pollack. *Nutrition, Stress and Aging*, New York, AMS Press, Inc., 1988.
15. Palm, J. Daniel. Diet Away Your Stress, Tension and Anxiety, New York, Doubleday and Company, Inc., 1976.
16. President's Council on Physical Fitness and Sports, *Physical Fitness Research Digest*, Series L, July, 1971.
17. Selye, Hans. Stress and Physical Activity, *Stress, The Official Journal of the International Institute of Stress and Its Affiliates*, Summer, 1981.
18. Walker, C. Eugene. *Learn to Relax, 13 Ways to Reduce Tension*, Englewood Cliffs, NJ, Prentice-Hall, Inc., 1975.

CHAPTER EIGHT

HOW NURSES CAN INDUCE THE RELAXATION RESPONSE TO REDUCE STRESS

R ELAX!!! How many times have you heard this expression? Although it has frequent usage as a means of telling a person to "take
it easy," or "slow down," more often than not those using the expression
are not aware of its real meaning. Most of us need some sort of relaxation in order to relieve the tensions encountered in daily living. The
purpose of this final chapter is to explore various facets of relaxation,
along with those kinds of conditions that tend to produce a relaxed state.
There are many procedures that can help improve a person's ability to
relax, and thus reduce stress. It should be borne in mind that what may
be satisfactory for one person may not necessarily be so for another.

The preceding chapter was concerned with general health practices
that can reduce stress. In this chapter the specific stress reduction techniques of *relaxation* is taken into account.

As mentioned previously, 69 percent of my nurse respondents indicated that they "engage in passive recreational activities," and included
among such activities were reading, listening to music, gardening and
needlework. These kinds of activities are more concerned with mental
diversion than they are with relaxation. What we are concerned with in
this chapter is relaxation as it pertains to muscular tension. It should be
recalled that 30 percent of the nurse respondents stated that they
engaged in such relaxation procedures.

THE MEANING OF RELAXATION

The reality of muscle fibers is that they have a response repertoire of
one. All they can do is contract and this is the response they make to the

103

electrochemical stimulation of impulses carried via the motor nerves. *Relaxation* is the removal of this stimulation.[3]

A relatively new term, *relaxation response*, has been coined by Herbert Benson.[2] This involves a number of bodily changes that occur in the organism when one experiences deep muscle relaxation. There is a response against "overstress," which brings on these bodily changes and brings the body back into what is a healthier balance. Thus, the purpose of any kind of relaxation technique should be to *induce the relaxation response*.

Some years ago, my friend, the late Arthur Steinhaus,[7] a notable physiologist, indicated that from the point of view of the physiologist, relaxation is sometimes considered as "zero activity," or as nearly zero as one can manage in the neuromuscular system. That is, it is a neuromuscular accomplishment that results in reduction, or possible complete absence of muscle tone in a part of, or in the entire body. It has been suggested that a primary value of relaxation lies in lowering of brain and spinal cord activity, resulting from a reduction of nerve impulses arising in muscle spindles and other sense endings in muscles, tendons, and joint structures.

The terms *relaxation, refreshment,* and *recreation* are often confused in their meaning. Although all of these factors are important to the well-being of the human organism, they should not be used interchangeably to mean the same thing. *Refreshment* is the result of an improved blood supply to the brain for "refreshment" from central fatigue and to the muscles for the disposition of their waste products. This explains in part why mild muscular activity is good for overcoming the fatigue of sitting quietly (seventh inning stretch) and for hastening recovery after strenuous exercise (an athlete continuing running for a short distance slowly after a race).

Recreation may be described as the experience from which a person emerges with the feeling of being "re-created." No single activity is sure to bring this experience to all members of a group, nor is there assurance that an activity will provide recreation again for a given person because it did so the last time. These are more the marks of a psychological than a physiological experience. An important essential requirement for a recreational activity is that it completely engross the individual; that is, it must engage his or her entire undivided attention. It is really escape from the disintegrating effects of distraction to the healing effect of totally integrated activity. Experiences that produce this effect may range from a hard game of tennis to the reading of a comic strip.

Some individuals consider recreation and relaxation to be one and the same thing, which is not the case. Recreation can be considered a type of mental diversion that can be helpful in relieving tension. Although mental and muscular tensions are interrelated, it is in the muscle that the tension state is manifested.

For many years recommendations have been made with regard to procedures individuals might apply in an effort to relax. Examples of some of these procedures are submitted in the ensuring discussions. In consideration of any technique designed to accomplish relaxation, one very important factor that needs to be taken into account is that learning to relax is a skill. That is, it is a skill based on the kinesthetic awareness of feelings of *tonus* (the normal degree of contraction present in most muscles, which keeps them always ready to function when needed). Unfortunately, it is a skill that very few of us practice — probably because we have little awareness of how to go about it.

One of the first steps in learning to relax is to experience tension. That is, one should be sensitive to tensions that exist in his or her body. This can be accomplished by voluntarily contracting a given muscle group, first very strongly and then less and less. Emphasis should be placed on detecting the signal of tension as the first step in "letting go" (relaxing).

You might wish to try the traditional experiment used to demonstrate this phenomenon. Raise one arm so that the palm of the hand is facing outward away from your face. Now, bend the wrist backward and try to point the fingers back toward your face and down toward the forearm. You should feel some *strain* at the wrist joint. You should also feel something else in the muscle and this is tension, which is due to the muscle contracting the hand backward. Now, flop the hand forward with the fingers pointing downward and you will have accomplished a *tension-relaxation cycle*.

As in the case of any skill, learning how to relax takes time and one should not expect to achieve complete satisfaction immediately. After one has identified a relaxation technique that he or she feels comfortable with, increased practice should eventually achieve satisfactory results.

PROGRESSIVE RELAXATION

The technique of progressive relaxation was developed by Edmund Jacobson many years ago. It is still the technique most often referred to in the literature and probably the one that has had the most widespread application. Twenty-two percent of the nurses in my survey used this technique. In this technique, the person concentrates on progressively relaxing one muscle group after another. The technique is based on the procedure of comparing the difference between tension and relaxation. That is, as previously mentioned, one senses the feeling of tension in order to get the feeling of relaxation.

It has already been said that learning to relax is a skill that you can develop in applying the principles of progressive relaxation. One of the first steps is to be able to identify the various muscle groups and how to tense them so that tension and relaxation can be experienced. However, before making suggestions on how to tense and relax the various muscle groups there are certain preliminary measures that need to be taken into account:

1. You must understand that this procedure takes time and like anything else, the more you practice the more proficient you should become with the skills.

2. Progressive relaxation is not the kind of thing to be done spontaneously, and you should be prepared to spend from 20 to 30 minutes daily in tensing-relaxing activities.

3. The particular time of day is important and this is pretty much an individual matter. Some recommendations suggest that progressive relaxation be practiced daily; sometime during the day and again in the evening before retiring. For many people this would be difficult unless one time period was set aside before going to the job in the morning. This might be a good possibility and might help a person to start the day relaxed.

4. It is important to find a suitable place to practice the tensing-relaxing activities. Again, this is an individual matter with some preferring a bed or couch and others a comfortable chair.

5. Consideration should be given to the amount of time a given muscle is tensed. You should be sure that you are able to feel the difference between tension and relaxation. This means that tension should be maintained from about four to not more than eight seconds.

6. Breathing is an important concomitant in tensing and relaxing muscles. To begin with, it is suggested that three or more deep breaths be taken and held for about five seconds. This will tend to make for better rhythm in breathing. Controlled breathing makes it easier to relax and it is most effective when it is done deeply and slowly. It is

ordinarily recommended that one should inhale deeply when the muscles are tensed and exhale slowly when "letting go." The reader is reminded that about 11 percent of the nurses in my survey used some sort of deep breathing to relieve stress.

How to Tense and Relax Various Muscles

Muscle groups may be identified in different ways. The classification given here consists of four different groups: (1) muscles of the head, face, tongue, and neck, (2) muscles of the trunk, (3) muscles of the upper extremities, and (4) muscles of the lower extremities.

Muscles of the Head, Face, Tongue, and Neck

There are two chief muscles of the head, the one covering the back of the head and the one covering the front of the skull. There are about 30 muscles of the face including the muscles of the orbit and eyelids, mastication, lips, tongue, and neck. Incidentally, it has been estimated that it takes 26 facial muscles to frown and a proportionately much smaller number to smile.

Muscles of this group may be tensed and relaxed as follows (relaxation is accomplished by "letting go" after tensing):

1. Raise your eyebrows by opening the eyes as wide as possible. You might wish to look into a mirror to see if you have formed wrinkles on the forehead.
2. Tense the muscles on either side of your nose like you were going to sneeze.
3. Dilate or flare out the nostrils.
4. Force an extended smile from "ear to ear" and at the same time clench your teeth.
5. Pull one corner of your mouth up and then the other corner up as in a "villainous sneer."
6. Draw your chin as close to your chest as possible.
7. Do the opposite of the above trying to draw your head back as close to your back as possible.

Muscles of the Trunk

Included in this group are the muscles of the back, chest, abdomen, and pelvis. Here are some ways to tense some of these muscles.

1. Bring your chest forward and at the same time put your shoulders

back with emphasis on bringing your shoulder blades as close together as possible.

2. Try to round your shoulders and bring them up to your ears at the
   same time as you try to bring your neck downward.
3. Give your shoulders a shrug trying to bring them up to your ears at
   the same time as you try to bring your neck downward.
4. Breathe deeply and hold it momentarily and then blow out the air
   from your lungs rapidly.
5. Draw in your stomach so that your chest is out beyond your stomach. Exert your stomach muscles by forcing out to make it look like
   you are fatter in that area than you are.

Muscles of the Upper Extremities

This group includes the muscles of the hands, forearms, upper arms,
and shoulders. A number of muscles situated in the trunk may be
grouped with the muscles of the upper extremities, their function being
to attach the upper limbs to the trunk and move the shoulders and arms.
In view of this there is some overlapping in muscle groups *two* and *three*.
Following are some ways to tense some of these muscles.

1. Clench the fist and then open the hand, extending the fingers as far
   as possible.
2. Raise one arm shoulder high and parallel to the floor. Bend at the
   elbow and bring the hand in toward the shoulder. Try to touch your
   shoulders while attempting to move the shoulder away from the
   hand. Flex your opposite biceps in the same manner.
3. Stretch one arm out to the side of the body and try to point the
   fingers backward toward the body. Do the same with the other
   arm.
4. Hold the arm out the same way as above but this time have the palm
   facing up and point the fingers inward toward the body. Do the
   same with the other arm.
5. Stretch one arm out to the side, clench the fist and roll the wrist
   around slowly. Do the same with the other arm.

Muscles of the Lower Extremities

This group includes muscles of the hips, thighs, legs, feet, and buttocks. Following are ways to tense some of these muscles.

1. Hold one leg out straight and point your toes as far forward as you
   can. Do the same thing with the other leg.

2. Do the same as above but point your toes as far backward as you can.
3. Turn each foot outward as far as you can and release. Do just the opposite by turning the foot inward as far as you can.
4. Try to draw the thigh muscles up so that you can see the form of the muscles.
5. Make your buttocks tense by pushing down if you are sitting in a chair. If you are lying down try to draw the muscles of the buttocks in close by attempting to force the cheeks together.

The above suggestions include several possibilities for tensing various muscles of the body. As you practice some of these, you will also discover other ways to tense and then let go. A word of caution might be that, in the early stages, you should be alert to the possibility of cramping certain muscles. This can happen particularly with those muscles that are not frequently used. This means that at the beginning you should proceed carefully. It might be a good idea to keep a record or diary of your sessions so that you can refer back to these experiences if this might be necessary. This will also help you get into each new session by reviewing your experiences in previous sessions.

Two other forms of relaxation will be taken into account here — *meditation* and *biofeedback*. Less than five percent of the nurse respondents indicated that they engaged in meditation to reduce stress; however, those that did use this technique reported great success with it and said that they would recommend it very highly to others. As far as biofeedback is concerned, about six percent of the nurses used this technique; however, a few of them reported that some aspect of biofeedback had been used in hospitals where they worked.

It is important that some attention be given to the underlying theories of progressive relaxation, meditation and biofeedback. In progressive relaxation, it is theorized that if the muscles of the body are relaxed, the mind in turn will be quieted. In the practice of meditation it is believed that if the mind is quieted, then other systems of the body will tend to be more readily stabilized. In biofeedback the theoretical basis tends to involve some sort of integration of progressive relaxation and meditation. It is believed that the brain has the potential for voluntary control over all the systems it monitors, and is affected by all of these systems. Thus, it is the intimacy of interaction between mind and body that has provided the mechanism through which one can learn voluntary control over biological activity.

It is interesting to note that in one study[5] nurses receiving either biofeedback training or progressive muscle relaxation (one hour daily for two weeks) reported significant improvements in ability to cope with stress compared to controls at three-month follow-up. However, in another study[1] it was reported that three hours of cognitive behavioral stress management training reduced anxiety among inexperienced burn unit nurses but *not* experienced ones. Also a stress "inoculation" treatment consisting of coping skills (time management, relaxation training, assertive skill building, cognitive restructuring), education, and exposure to simulated stressors produced significant improvements in stress responses and complaints among acute care RNs after four weeks and at four-month follow-up.[8] The treatment was superior to education and coping alone, education and exposure alone, education only, or no treatment.

In summary, all of the techniques — progressive relaxation, meditation, and biofeedback — are concerned with mind-body interactions, and all of them are designed to induce the relaxation response mentioned at the beginning of the chapter.

MEDITATION

The Eastern art of meditation dates back more than 2000 years. Until recently, this ancient art has been encumbered with religious as well as cultural connotations. In the 1960s, counter cultures began using it as a route to a more natural means of living and relaxing. Today, persons from all walks of life can be counted among the untold numbers around the world who practice and realize the positive effects that meditation can have upon the human mind and body.

It has been asserted by Kenneth Pelletier[6] that meditation should be defined as an experimental exercise involving an individual's actual attention, not belief-systems or other cognitive processes, and that it should not be confused with prolonged, self-induced lethargy. The nervous system needs intensity and variety of external stimulation to maintain proper functioning.

Although there are many meditation techniques, *concentration* is a very essential factor contributing to success. The mind's natural flow from one idea to another is quieted by the individual's concentration. Lowering mental activity may be an easy task, but almost total elimination of scattered thoughts takes a great deal of time and practice on the part of the meditator.

The question sometimes raised is, "Are sleep and meditation the same thing"? Sleep has been likened to meditation, as both are hypometabolic states; that is, restful states where the body experiences decreased metabolism. But meditation is not a form of sleep. Although some similar psychological changes have been found in sleep and meditation, they are not the same and one is not a substitute for the other. In this regard, it is interesting that various studies have shown that meditation may restore more energy than sleep.

There have been countless positive pronouncements about meditation from some of the most notable scientists of modern times, who spend a good portion of their time studying about stress. However, it has been in relatively recent years only that the scientific community has uncovered many of the positive effects that the repeated practice of meditation has upon those who are stress ridden. Various scientific studies have shown that meditation can actually decrease the possibilities of an individual contracting stress-related disorders, and that meditators have a much faster recovery rate when exposed to a stressful situation than nonmeditators. Specifically, from a physiological point of view it has been found that meditation decreases the body's metabolic rate, with the following decreases in bodily function involved: (1) oxygen consumption, (2) breathing rate, (3) heart rate and blood pressure, (4) sympathetic nervous system activity, and (5) blood lactate (a chemical produced in the body during stressful encounters). Also meditation tends to increase the physiological stability of those who practice it, as well as to reduce anxiety.[2]

Although there are many meditation techniques, research tends to show that one technique is about as good as another for improving the way one handles stress. Of the various types of meditation, transcendental meditation (TM) is by far the best known. It was introduced in the United States many years ago by Mararishi Mahesh Yogi. It is believed that he used the term *transcendental* (a literal meaning of which is "going beyond") to indicate that it projects one beyond the level of a wakeful experience to a state of profound rest along with heightened alertness.

TM involves the repetition of a *mantra* (a word or specific sound) for 15 to 20 minutes daily with the meditator in a relaxed position with closed eyes. Almost without exception those who have practiced TM attest to its positive effects. While other forms of meditation may have specific procedures, it is safe to say that most derive in some way from basic TM.

A Procedure for Meditating

The description presented here is a procedure for meditating that I have found has met with personal success. In addition, many of my students — nurses as well as others — have reported success with its use. However, it should be remembered that it is pretty much an individual matter, and what may be successful for one person may not necessarily be successful for another.

To begin with, there are certain basic considerations that should be taken into account. The following descriptive list of these considerations is general in nature, and the reader can make his or her own specific application as best fits individual needs and interests.

1. *Locate a quiet place and assume a comfortable position.* The importance of a quiet environment should be obvious since concentration is facilitated in a tranquil surrounding. The question of the position one may assume for meditation is an individual matter. However, when it is suggested that one assume a comfortable position, this might be amended by, "but not too comfortable." The reason for this is that if one is too comfortable there is the possibility of falling asleep, and this, of course, would defeat the purpose of meditation. This is a reason why one should consider not taking a lying position while meditating.

   A position might be taken where there is some latitude for "swaying." This can provide for a comfortable posture and, at the same time, guard against the individual's "falling into dreamland." The main consideration is that the person be in a comfortable enough position to remain this way for a period of at least 15 minutes or so. One such position would be where you sit on the floor with legs crossed and the back straight and resting on the legs and buttocks. Your head should be erect and the hands resting in the lap. If you prefer to sit in a chair rather than on the floor, select a chair with a straight back. You need to be the judge of comfort, and, thus, you should select a position where you feel you are able to concentrate and remain in this position for a period of time.

2. *Focus your concentration.* As mentioned before, concentration is the essential key to successful meditation. If you focus on one specific thing, such as an object or sound or a personal feeling, it is less likely that your thoughts will be distracted. You might want to consider focusing on such things as a fantasy trip, reexperiencing a trip

already taken, a place that has not been visited, or a certain sound or chant.

3. *Use of a nonsense word or phrase.* Some techniques of meditation, such as the popular TM, involve the chanting of a particular word (mantra) as one meditates. While the mantra is important for the meditator, I refer to it as a nonsense word because it should be devoid of any connotation that would send one thinking in many directions. This, of course, would hinder concentration, so a nonsense word would perhaps be most effective.

4. *Be aware of natural breathing rhythm.* The importance of natural breathing rhythm should not be underestimated. In fact, some clinical psychologists recommend this as a means of concentrating. That is, one can count the number of time he or she inhales and exhales, and this in itself is a relaxing mental activity.

5. *The time for meditation.* Since meditation is an activity to quiet the mind it is strongly recommended that the practice not be undertaken immediately upon arriving home from work. At this time, the mind may be in a very active state of reviewing the day's activities. My own personal experience suggests a 15 to 20 minute period in the morning, and another such period in the evening preferably before dinner, or possibly two hours after dinner. Experience has shown that food in the gastrointestinal tract appears to interfere with effective meditation. Therefore, if a person feels hungry or thirsty, a drink and small snack should be taken about one hour before meditating.[4]

With the above basic considerations in mind you should be ready to experiment. To begin with, assume a comfortable position in a quiet place with as passive an attitude as possible. Try to dismiss all wandering thoughts from your mind and concentrate on a relaxed body while keeping the eyes closed. When feeling fairly relaxed, the repetition of the nonsense word or phrase can begin. This can be repeated orally or silently. Personally, I have good success repeating it silently; that is, through the mind. Repeat your chosen word or phrase in this manner over and over, keeping the mind clear of any passing thoughts. At first, this may be very difficult, but with practice it becomes easier.

After a period of about 15 or 20 minutes have passed, discontinue repetition of the word or phrase. Become aware of your relaxed body once again. Give yourself a few moments before moving as your body will need to readjust. For successful prolonged results one might consider continuing the practice two times daily for 15 or 20 minute sessions.

If you have difficulty trying to meditate on your own, it is possible to seek the services of an experienced meditator for assistance and supervision. The recent widespread popularity of meditation has been accompanied by the establishment of meditation centers for instruction in some communities.

BIOFEEDBACK

In the discussion of biofeedback, it should be made luminously clear that we are dealing with a complex and complicated subject. It will be the purpose to discuss this phenomenon in terms of what it is supposed to be and what it is supposed to do. It should be borne in mind that, at least in the early stages, biofeedback training (BFT), an important factor is that it take place under qualified supervision. This means that should you wish to pursue an interest in and eventually participate in BFT, you should seek the services of one trained in this area. (Incidentally, as nurses know, many hospitals engage in biofeedback activity. You might wish to check this out in your own institution.)

The Meaning of Biofeedback

The term *feedback* has been used in various frames of reference. It may have been used originally in engineering in connection with control systems that involve feedback procedures. These feedback control systems make adjustments to environmental changes, such as the case of your thermostat controlling temperature levels in your home.

Biofeedback helps people to self-regulate; gain more control over their lives. Successful biofeedback self-regulation in one area of life can often lead to improvement in other areas, including nutrition, exercise, quality of relationships, and lifestyle. Increased self-confidence and ability to transfer the learning are among the factors that make this possible.

Biofeedback Instrumentation

We are all aware of the fact that the human body itself is a complicated and complex biofeedback instrument, which alerts us to certain internal activity. However, many students of the subject feel that there is still a need for sensitive instruments to monitor physiological and psychological reactivity. Following is a brief discussion of some of these instruments.

Electromyograph (EMG)

Electromyography is the recording of electric phenomena occurring in muscles during contraction. Needle or skin electrodes are used and connected with an oscilloscope so that action potentials may be viewed and recorded (the oscilloscope is an instrument that visually displays an electrical wave on a florescent screen). Before the electromyograph was available, guesswork ordinarily had to be used to try to determine the participation of the muscles in movement. When a muscle is completely relaxed or inactive, it has no electric potential; however, when it is engaged in contraction, current appears.

It is believed that EMG training can produce deep muscle relaxation and relieve tension. A person gets the feedback by seeing a dial or hearing a sound from the machine, and he or she knows immediately the extent to which certain muscles may be relaxed or tensed. A muscle frequently used in EMG training for research and other purposes is the *frontalis* located in the front of the head. Another important aspect of EMG is that which is concerned with retraining a person following an injury, or disease when there is a need to observe small increments of gain in function of a muscle.

Feedback Thermometers

The obvious purpose of feedback thermometers is to record body temperatures, Ordinarily, a thermistor is attached to the hands or the fingers. This highly sensitive instrument shows very small increments of degrees of temperature change so that the person receives the information with a visual or auditory signal. This kind of feedback instrumentation has been recommended for such purposes as reduction of stress and anxiety and autonomic nervous system relaxation.

Electroencephalograph (EEG)

The purpose of this instrument is to record amplitude and frequency of brain waves, and it has been used in research for many years. It has also been used with success to diagnose certain clinical diseases. In addition, EEG feedback has found use in psychotherapy, and in reducing stress as well as pain.

An interesting relatively recent horizon for EEG feedback is how it might be involved in creativity and learning. In fact, some individuals involved in creative activity have indicated that they can emerge from the EEG *theta* state with answers to problems that they previously were unable to solve. The theta waves are ordinarily recorded when a person is in a state of drowsiness or actually falling asleep. It is perhaps for this reason that this condition has been referred to by some as "sleep learning." Since it is a state just before sleep, others refer to it as the twilight period or *twilight learning*.

Galvanic Skin Response (GSR)

There are several different kinds of GSR instruments used to measure changes in electrical resistance of the skin to detect emotional arousal. The instrument reacts in proportion to the amount of perspiration one emits and the person is informed of the changes in electrical resistance by an auditory or visual signal. One aspect of GSR is concerned with the use of the polygraph or lie detector, which is supposed to record a response that is concerned with lying, GSR feedback is oftentimes recommended for use of relaxation, reducing tension, improvement of ability to sleep, or for emotional control.

In general, the purpose of the biofeedback machinery is to provide accurate and reliable data that will increase one's influence of this action of his body. This information should be useful in inspiring a person to take an active self-interest in his own well-being. After such information is received, if it has been obtained under the supervision of a qualified person, there may be a given number of sessions arranged for consultation and training. Perhaps the ultimate objective is for the individual to be able to gain control over his or her own autonomic nervous system.

At the present time it is difficult to determine unequivocally what the future of biofeedback may be. Without question, it has influenced our way of thinking with reference to a person being able to possibly control his physiological functions. In view of this, perhaps one of its foremost contributions is that it creates in an individual a feeling of his own responsibility for his personal well-being.

All of the recommendations made here have met with varying degrees of success with persons who have practiced them. Individual differences indicate that one person may find more success than another with given procedures. One of the most important factors to take into account is that stress management is pretty much an individual matter.

Table 6
Percent of Nurses Using Relaxation Techniques

Technique	Percent Using
Progressive Relaxation	22%
Biofeedback	6%
Meditation	4%

With practice, most of you will have some degree of success in your attempts to manage your own stressful conditions. Above all, a positive attitude toward life in general is an essential prerequisite for any kind of stress management program that is undertaken.

REFERENCES

1. Baeyer, Carl von and L. Krause. Effectiveness of Stress Management Training for Nurses Working in a Burn Treatment Unit, *International Journal of Psychiatry in Medicine,* 13, 1983.
2. Benson, Herbert. *The Relaxation Response,* New York, William Morrow, 1985.
3. Brown, Barbara B. *Stress and the Art of Biofeedback,* New York, Bantam Books, 1978.
4. Morse, Donald and Robert Pollack. *Nutrition, Stress and Aging,* New York, AMS Press, Inc., 1988.
5. Murphy, L. A Comparison of Relaxation Methods for Reducing Stress in Nursing Personnel, *Human Factors,* 25, 1983.
6. Pelletier, Kenneth R. *Mind as Healer Mind as Slayer,* New York, Dell, 1977.
7. Steinhaus, Arthur. *Toward an Understanding of Health and Physical Education,* Dubuque, Iowa, Wm. C. Brown, 1963.
8. West, D.J., J.J. Horan, and P.A. Games. Component Analysis of Occupational Stress Inoculation Applied to Registered Nurses in an Acute Hospital Setting, *Journal of Counseling Psychology,* 31, 1984.

BIBLIOGRAPHY

Alonso, R.C., J.A. Alutto, and L.G. Hrebiniak. Job Tensions Among Hospital Employed Nurses, *Supervisor Nurse*, 3, 1972.

Bailey, J.T. and D.D. Walker. Rx for Stress: One Hospital's Approach, *Supervisory Management*, 27, 1982.

Baldwin, A. and J.T. Bailey. Work-Site Interventions for Stress Reduction, *Journal of Nursing Education*, 10, 1980.

Banks, J. Stress Management for Black Nurses, *Journal of Black Nurses Association*, Spring, 1986.

Beaver, R.C., E.S. Sharp, and G.A. Cotsonis. Burnout Experienced by Nurse Midwives, *Journal of Nurse Midwife*, 31, 1986.

Blanks, C.D. and G. Giovinco. Stress/Burnout Indicators of Concern Across Clinical Areas of Nursing, *Florida Nurse*, 34, 1986.

Bourbonnais, F.F. and A. Bauman. Stress and Rapid Decision Making in Nursing: An Administrative Challenge, *Nurse Adm Quarterly*, 9, 1985.

Brosnan, J. and M. Johnston. Stressed by Satisfied: Organizational Change in Ambulatory Care, *Journal of Nursing Administration*, October 1980.

Calhoun, G.L. Hospitals Are High-Stress Employers, Hospitals, June, 1980.

Campbell, C. Stress Survey, Disturbing Findings, *Nurse Mirror*, June, 1985.

Cassem, N.H. and T.P. Hacket. Stress on the Nurse and Therapist in the Intensive-Care Unit and the Coronary Care Unit, *Heart and Lung*, 4, 1975.

Castledine, G. When the Pressure Gets Too Much, *Nursing Times*, May, 1985.

Cavagnaro, M.A. A Comparison Study of Stress Factors as They Affect CRNAs. *AANA Journal*, June, 1983.

Cray, B. Nurses in Society: Led by Stress, *Nurse Mirror*, June, 1983.

Davis, A.J. Stress, *American Journal of Nursing*, March, 1984.

Davis, M. Assessing Nurses. Stress in Assessment, *Nursing Times*, July 30-August 5, 1986.

Duxbury, M.L., G.D. Armstrong, D.J. Drew, and S.J. Henly. Head Nurse Leadership Style With Staff Nurse Burnout and Job Satisfaction in Neonatal Intensive Care Units, *Nursing Research*, 33, 1984.

Evison, R. Self-Help in Preventing Stress Build-Up, *Professional Nurse*, March, 1986.

Faulconer, D.R. and V.B. Goldman. On the Scene: Mount Sinai Medical Center of Greater Miami, Managerial Stress, *Nursing Adm Quarterly*, Winter, 1983.

Fawzy, F.I., D.K. Wellisch, R.O. Pasnau, and B. Leibowitz. Preventing Nursing Burnout: A Challenge for Liason Psychiatry, *General Hospital Psychiatry*, July, 1983.

Gardner, D., Z. Parzen, and N. Stewart. The Nurse's Dilemma: Mediating Stress in Critical Care Units, *Heart and Lung,* September, 1980.

Gillis, A. Coping and Controlling: A Problem for Nursing, *Canadian Journal of Psychiatric Nursing,* April-June, 1984.

Gribbins, R.E. and R.E. Marshall. Stress and Coping Strategies of Nurse Manager in the NICU, *American Journal of Perinatol,* April, 1984.

Haack, M. and J.W. Jones. Diagnosing Burnout, Using Projective Drawings, *Journal of Psychosocial Nurse in Mental Health Service,* July, 1983.

Haddad, A.M. Caring for Yourself Comes First, *RN,* June, 1984.

Harris, P.L. Burnout in Nursing Administration, *Nursing Adm Quarterly,* Spring, 1984.

Hartl, D.E. Stress Management and the Nurse, *Advanced Nursing Science,* January, 1979.

Hsia, L. Burnout, *Journal of Nurse Midwife,* May-June, 1986.

Henry, B.M. and L.E. Moody. Energize With Laughter, *Nursing Success Today,* January, 1985.

Holyoke, A. Burnout, or Cop Out? *Diabetes Education,* Fall, 1984.

Ivesson-Eveson, J. Banishing the Burnout Syndrome, *Nurse Mirror,* May, 1983.

Jacobson, S. Stressful Situations for Neonatal Intensive Care Unit Nurses, *American Journal Maternal Child Nursing,* March, 1978.

Jalorviec, A. and M.J. Powers. Stress and Coping in Hypertensive and Emergency Patients, *Nursing Research,* October, 1981.

Johnson, M.N. Anxiety-Stress and the Effects on Disclosure Between Nurses and Patients, *Advanced Nursing Science,* January, 1979.

Kovecses, J. Burnout Doesn't Have to Happen, *Nurse,* November, 1980.

Kramer, M. *Reality Shock: Why Nurses Leave Nursing,* St. Louis, Mosby, 1974.

Lavandero, R. Nurse Burnout: What Can We Learn? *The Journal of Nursing Administration,* 12, 1981.

Leatt, P. and R. Schneck. Perceptions of Stress by Nurses in Different Specialties: Some Implications for Nursing Administrators, *Nurs Pap,* Winter, 1983.

Leatt, P. and R. Schneck. Differences in Stress Perceived by Headnurses Across Nursing Specialties in Hospitals, *Journal of Advanced Nursing,* 5, 1980.

Levenstein, A. Evaluating the Stressors in Your Life, Art and Science of Management, *Nurse Management,* August, 1986.

Livingston, M. and H. Livingston, Emotional Distress in Nurses at Work, *British Journal of Medical Psychology,* September, 1984.

Marchetti, J. Role Change, Stress . . . and You! Moving up From Clinical Nurse to Management, *Nursing Success Today,* March, 1985.

Marshall, J. *Stress Amongst Nurses,* in C.L. Cooper and R. Payne (eds.), New York, Wiley, 1978.

Moore, J.G. Burnout—A New Name for an Old Problem, *Midwife Health Visiting Community Nurse,* September, 1983.

Morrison, I. The Plight of the District Nurse, *Nursing Times,* January, 1984.

Morton-Cooper, A. Nurses in Trouble, *Nurse Mirror,* December, 1984.

Numeroff, R.E. and M.N. Abrams. Sources of Stress Among Nurses: An Empirical Investigation, *Journal of Human Stress,* 10, 1984.

Nurses in Society: Burnout, *Nurse Mirror,* February, 1984.

O'Neill, K. Stress, Substance Use and the Nurse, *Lamp,* December, 1984.

Parkes, K.R. Occupational Stress Among Student Nurses: A Natural Experiment, *Journal of Applied Psychology,* 67, 1982.

Patrick, P.K. Organizational Burnout Program, *Journal of Nursing Administration,* June, 1984.

Pines, A.M. and A.D. Kanner. Nurses' Burnout: Lack of Positive Conditions and Presence of Negative Conditions as Two Independent Sources of Stress, *Journal of Psychosocial Nursing and Mental Health Services,* 20, 1982.

Poole, C.J. Brightly Burning Nurses Revisited, *Nurse Management,* April, 1985.

Rapson, M.F. Strategies for Coping With Role Stress, *Nurse Pract,* May, 1983.

Schmidt, C. Emotional Stress in the NICU, *P/N,* January, 1977.

Scully, R. Stress in the Nurse, *American Journal of Nursing,* 80, 1980.

Shubin, B. Burnout: The Professional Hazard You Face in Nursing, *Nurse,* August, 1978.

Stehle, J.L. Critical Care Nursing Stress: The Findings Revisited, *Nursing Research,* 30, 1981.

Stillman, S.M. and B.L. Strasser. Helping Critical Care Nurses With Work-Related Stress, *Journal of Nursing Administration,* October, 1980.

Storlie, F. Burnout: The Elaboration of a Concept, *American Journal of Nursing,* February, 1979.

Stress Survey, In Their Own Words, *Nurse Mirror,* June, 1985.

Sutterly, D.C. Stress Management: Grazing the Clinical Turf, *Holistic Nursing Practice,* November, 1986.

Tompkins, F.D. and L. Huckabay. Management Stress and Burnout, *Nursing Adm Quarterly,* Spring, 1984.

Ulberg, K. Burned Out: Should a Battle-Weary Nurse Endure—or Find Another Job? *Journal of Christian Nursing,* Summer, 1986.

Vousden, M. Taking the Strain, *Nurse Mirror,* August, 1985.

Wandelt, M., P. Pierce, and R. Widdowson. Why Nurses Leave Nursing and What Can Be Done About It, *American Journal of Nursing,* 81, 1981.

Weiner, M.F., T. Caldwell, and J. Tyson. Stresses and Coping in ICU Nursing: Why Support Groups Fail, *General Hospital Psychiatry,* September, 1983.

White, C.H. Where Have All the Nurses Gone—and Why? *Hospitals,* 54, 1980.

Wilson, J. Why Nurses Leave Nursing, *Canadian Nurse,* March, 1987.

Yasko, J.M. Variables Which Predict Burnout Experienced by Oncology Clinical Nurse Specialists, *Cancer Nursing,* April, 1983.

INDEX

123